Enjoy Optimal Health

98 Health Tips from a Family Doctor

Greg Feinsinger, M.D.

This book contains advice and information relating to health care. It should be used to supplement but not replace advice from trained medical professionals, who should be consulted regarding your specific situation. If you have symptoms that require a workup, diagnosis, and treatment plan, you should consult a competent physician or other trained health care provider. Neither the author nor the publisher shall be liable or responsible for any loss or damage allegedly arising from any information in this book.

ISBN: 978-1790821310

Library of Congress Control Number: 2019931624

Light of the Moon, Inc. - Publishing Division
Book Design/Production/Consulting
Carbondale, Colorado
www.lightofthemooninc.com

Praise for Dr. Feinsinger's work

I have had high blood pressure for years, and in June, 2016, had quadruple bypass surgery. I saw Dr. Feinsinger for one of his free consultations in March, 2018 and the plant-based diet he put me on helped me lose weight and get control of my blood pressure, cholesterol, and heart disease.   ~ J.T.

• • •

Several years ago I was diagnosed with breast cancer, which spread to my lymph nodes. After finishing radiation and chemotherapy, I wanted to clean up my diet—in particular I wanted food without antibiotics and growth hormones that could stimulate cancer cells. My husband was very supportive of going plant-based, and together we have been eating (and enjoying) a vegan diet for 10 years—and no cancer recurrence. I appreciate what Dr. Feinsinger is doing to spread the word about the power of food to people in the Roaring Fork Valley and beyond.   ~ L.F., D.O.

• • •

I was diagnosed with a 40-60% blockage in a coronary artery 5 years ago. Under Dr. Feinsinger's guidance, I went on a plant-based diet, which stopped the progression of my heart disease.   ~ E.P.

• • •

After my first heart attack, second angioplasty, and a pulmonary embolism, I looked for an alternative to what seemed like a future lifetime of invasive procedures. I asked my cardiologist about nutritional therapies and was told he know nothing about them but "good luck." A friend recommended that I see Dr. Feinsinger, who guided me towards a whole food, plant-based diet after explaining the science that supported this. My weight is now ideal, and my cholesterol has plummeted. Best of all, my previous, persistent angina pains have essentially resolved.   ~ P.T.

DEDICATION

This book is dedicated to my wife of fifty-two years, Kathy, who has many talents, including being a great cook. She urged me to read *The China Study* years ago, which changed our lives. Kathy has made our plant-based journey easy, pleasurable, and tasty.

TABLE OF CONTENTS

Diet—what we should avoid for optimal health

Diet, what we should be eating and drinking daily

Dopamine

Environment

Exercise

INTRODUCTION

At the University of Colorado School of Medicine in the 1960s, we learned that health was all about pills and procedures. We learned nothing about the power of food, and very little about prevention. When I attended my fiftieth medical school reunion, members of the graduating class of 2018 told me that things haven't changed.

In 2003, I found out that essentially all heart attacks—the number one cause of death in America—can be prevented, but that this doesn't happen due to money-driven inertia. We don't have a health care system, but rather we have a disease management system: we wait until diseases occur and then spend a lot of money and effort trying to manage them. In 2003 I started the Center for Heart Attack, Stroke and Diabetes Prevention at Glenwood Medical Associates, a multi-specialty group in Glenwood Springs, Colorado, where I practiced family medicine for forty-two years.

Heart attack prevention ended up being a large part of my practice. However, I still knew little about nutrition—until around 2010, on the advice of a nurse practitioner friend, my wife read *The China Study,* and urged me to read it. This study found that the people in China who were too poor to afford to eat animal protein were not afflicted by the chronic diseases that people on Western diets suffer and die from—obesity, hypertension, high cholesterol, heart attacks, and strokes, diabetes, dementia, inflammatory and autoimmune diseases, osteoporosis, macular degeneration, and many kinds of cancer (especially breast, colon, and prostate).

We found the China Study information so compelling that we immediately went on a plant-based, whole (unprocessed) food diet with no salt, sugar, or added oil. In a month I lost twelve pounds and ever since then have weighed what I did when I graduated from high school in 1959. The pre-diabetes and hypertension for which I was being medicated went away, and I was able to cut way back on my cholesterol medication. Furthermore, my athletic performance improved—I was able to beat people my age in running and Nordic ski races whom I hadn't beaten before.

I started telling my patients about plant-based nutrition and many of them complied, with amazing results—more improvement in their weight, blood pressure, blood sugar, and cholesterol than with any medication I had prescribed. And, they all felt better.

INTRODUCTION

This book is a compilation of ninety-eight of the weekly health columns I have written for the Glenwood *Post Independent* since I retired in 2015. The goal of the columns and this book is to enable readers to control their own health destiny.

I would like to thank my mentor in heart attack prevention for the past fifteen years, Brad Bale, M.D., co-author of *Beat the Heart Attack Gene*. Thank you to the giants in plant-based nutrition, especially T. Colin Campbell, PhD, Caldwell Esselstyn, M.D., Joel Fuhrman, M.D., Michael Greger, M.D., Dean Ornish, M.D., and Neal Barnard, M.D. Much of the information on these pages was derived from their research and writings, and I have tried to credit them when appropriate.

Martin Oswald, chef-owner of the Pyramid Bistro in Aspen deserves our gratitude for teaching us all how tasty plant-based food can be. Thank you to Peter Goldstein, of the website *Hippocrates Docs* and his program Just 1 Thing 4 Health, who is a colleague in promoting plant-based nutrition—without his perseverance and I.T. expertise, this book would not have been possible. Thank you to Rita Marsh, who through her non-profit Davi Nikent has been supportive of my endeavors. Finally, thank you to my oldest daughter, Christi Vogt, who has the talent and expertise to promote healthy living.

Greg Feinsinger, M.D., 2018

"Let food be thy medicine and
let medicine be thy food."

– Hippocrates,
the father of clinical medicine

WHEN IT COMES TO OUR HEALTH, WHAT DO WE WANT?

Here's what most people want when it comes to their health:
- Live to a ripe old age.
- Have a good quality of life until hours—or, at most, days—before they die, rather than the slow downhill course so many Americans have starting in their fifties or sixties.
- Have eyesight, normal mobility, and an intact brain until they die.
- Maintain their independence versus being institutionalized in a nursing home or assisted living.

What do most people die from in this country? In order of frequency, the top three causes of death are:
- Cardiovascular disease (heart attacks and strokes caused by atherosclerosis)
- Cancer
- Complications from our medical system (For example: side effects from prescription drugs, hospital-acquired infections, errors by doctors and other health care providers, mistakes that occur in hospitals. A recent Johns Hopkins University study found that more than 250,000 deaths a year were caused by mistakes by the American health care system.)

What are the main causes of disability?
- Strokes–which often leave victims paralyzed and/or unable to speak
- Complications of diabetes such as blindness, cardiovascular disease, kidney failure, neuropathy (pain and numbness in legs and feet that can lead to amputation)
- Mobility problems, often related to obesity
- Dementia, including Alzheimer's

Lifestyle modification, particularly daily exercise and a plant-based, whole (unprocessed) diet with no sugar, salt, and added oil have been shown to prevent most of the chronic diseases Americans suffer and die from: obesity, hypertension, high cholesterol, cardiovascular disease, type 2 diabetes, inflammatory diseases such as rheumatoid arthritis, auto-immune diseases such as M.S., dementia including Alzheimer's, and many forms of cancer. This lifestyle modification has also been shown to reverse many of these conditions if already present.

The goal of these health tips is to empower people to take control of their own health destiny. Of course, there are no 100 percent guarantees in life. A cartoon in the *New Yorker* magazine had a drawing of a gravestone with the inscription "I can't believe I ate all that kale for nothing." But if you want to live a long life of good quality, it would be wise to stack the deck in your favor. As Kim Williams, M.D., current president of the American College of Cardiology said when asked why he went plant-based, "I don't mind dying so much but I don't want it to be my fault."

Plant-based nutrition can be tasty. Some good cookbooks are:
- *The Oh She Glows Cookbook*
- *Isa Does It*
- *Thug Kitchen*
- *How Not to Die Cookbook*
- *Forks Over Knives Cookbook*
- *Vegan Richa's Indian Kitchen*
- *Simply Delicious*

"Two minutes from lips to hips."

- Joel Fuhrman, M.D.,

(Referring to the rapidity with which added oils
are absorbed into the blood stream and deposited as fat.)

PREVENTING ALZHEIMER'S DISEASE

One of the diseases that older people fear the most is Alzheimer's, first described in 1906 by the German physician Alois Alzheimer. An autopsy on his first dementia patient showed amyloid plaques and protein tangles in the brain, plus atherosclerosis of the cerebral (brain) arteries. Alzheimer's accounts for 60–70 percent of dementia, with conditions such as multiple small strokes accounting for the rest. The first symptom of Alzheimer's is short-term memory loss, and additional neuro-psychiatric symptoms appear with time.

As is often the case in our pharmaceutical-centric medical culture, patients and physicians are waiting for a magic pill to prevent or reverse the disease, even though reversal is probably unrealistic because once brain damage occurs it is usually irreversible. Like so many other maladies in Western societies, the way to prevent Alzheimer's is a change in lifestyle, particularly what we eat. Here is a summary of what we currently know about this disease, based on Dr. Michael Greger's book *How Not to Die* and his website *nutritionfacts.org*.

- The risk factors for Alzheimer's are the same as for atherosclerosis (hardening of the arteries): hypertension, high cholesterol, smoking, diabetes, inflammation, sedentary lifestyle. Alzheimer's patients who have their cardiovascular risk factors treated aggressively have slower mental decline.
- The brains of Alzheimer's patients have more cholesterol than those of normal people, and Alzheimer's might prove to be a vascular disease. Cholesterol seeds the clumping of amyloid plaque. High cholesterol in middle age triples the risk of Alzheimer's.
- Fifteen percent of the U.S. population have the ApoE4 gene, which makes the protein that carries cholesterol to the brain. One copy of ApoE4 triples the risk of Alzheimer's—2 copies of this gene (one from each parent) increases Alzheimer's by nine-fold. But while "genetics loads the gun, environment pulls the trigger." Nigeria has the highest incidence of the ApoE4 gene, but a very low incidence of Alzheimer's due to their plant-based, whole food (unprocessed) diet. (When Nigerians eat the Standard American Diet—S.A.D.— the ApoE4 gene is turned on and they tend to get Alzheimer's.)
- The lowest rate of Alzheimer's is in rural India—thought to be due to their plant-based diet and presence of turmeric in the curry they eat (they average

1/4 tsp. of turmeric a day).

- Phytonutrients (phyto = plant) such as antioxidants help prevent Alzheimer's, and are particularly abundant in intensely-colored plants such as greens and berries; and in intensely-flavored food such as herbs and spices.
- The Harvard Women's Health Study found that higher saturated fat intake from dairy, meat, and processed foods was associated with cognitive decline.
- Heavy metals such as iron and copper are concentrated in amyloid plaque and tangles, but only in people on an animal-based diet. Avoid supplements such as multivitamin and mineral pills that contain these elements. Also, cook with ceramic, stainless steel, or glass cookware and avoid copper pans and iron skillets. Although not 100 percent proven, aluminum might be a problem too, so to be safe avoid aluminum foil and cookware.
- Saffron has been used in traditional Persian medicine for cognitive decline. Thirty mg. a day works just as well as the current Alzheimer's drugs such as Na-menda. (The current drugs are minimally effective and often have side ef-fects—which saffron doesn't.)
- In a small study, people with mild to moderate Alzheimer's symptoms were given 1 tsp. of turmeric a day and the symptoms resolved—which is unheard of.
- Regular exercise has clearly been shown to help prevent and even improve Alzheimer's.

In summary, if you're concerned about maintaining normal brain function as you age, don't wait for the pharmaceutical industry to come up with a magic bullet, which may or may not ever happen (even if it does, it will likely be expensive and have side effects). Instead, do what the journal *Neurobiology of Aging* recommended in 2014: "Vegetables, legumes (beans, peas, and lentils), fruits, and whole grains should replace meats and dairy products as primary staples of the diet."

ALZHEIMER'S

ALZHEIMER'S: HOW INADEQUATE SLEEP, CERTAIN MEDICATIONS, AND CERTAIN MEDICAL CONDITIONS CAN ADVERSELY AFFECT YOUR BRAIN

This health tip is about the memory-robbing disease Alzheimer's, based on Dr. Neal Barnard's book *Power Foods For The Brain, An Effective 3-Step Plan to Protect Your Mind and Strengthen Your Memory.*

SLEEP

We all have experienced brain fog after a night of inadequate sleep. Sleep is critical for optimal brain function. In the first half of the night we consolidate memories of facts and events. In the second half of the night, when REM (rapid eye movement) predominates, we integrate memories related to new skills and to emotions. The production of amyloid brain plaque associated with Alzheimer's is higher during the day than it is during restful sleep at night. Following are factors that adversely affect sleep:

- Caffeine: The half-life of caffeine is about 6 hours. If you have a cup of coffee at 8 a.m., a quarter of the caffeine is still in your bloodstream at 8 p.m.
- Alcohol helps you fall asleep, but the aldehydes that form from alcohol stimulate you, causing early-morning awakening.
- High protein foods in the evening interfere with sleep by blocking serotonin production.
- Prostate problems in aging men interrupt sleep by causing urination frequency.
- Sleep apnea, both obstructive and central (the latter is related to living at altitude). Anyone with signs suggestive of dementia should have an overnight pulse oximetry to screen for sleep apnea.

MEDICATIONS

- Prescription sleep meds such as Ambien, Halcion, and Sonata can cause mental fogginess and memory issues.
- Over-the-counter sleep aids such as Benadryl, Sominex, and Unisom can do the same thing.

- Anti-histamines used for allergies (e.g. diphenhydramine, chlorpheniramine) and to treat cold symptoms (e.g. Nyquil) can adversely affect brain function.
- Certain anti-depressants can cause brain fog, such Elavil, Tofranil, Effexor, Prozac, and Paxil.
- Anti-anxiety drugs such as Valium, Ativan, and Xanax can interfere with memory and thinking.
- Narcotic pain pills, such as Percodan and Vicodin can also cause brain fog.
- Beta blockers, sometimes used for hypertension and heart irregularities, such as propranolol and atenolol also cause brain fog.
- Statins can rarely cause brain fog, but on the other hand they lower high cholesterol that left untreated raises the risk of dementia.

MEDICAL CONDITIONS

- Depression and anxiety can cause sleep, thinking, and memory difficulties. Pseudo-dementia occurs in elderly people who appear to have dementia but are actually just depressed.
- Coronary bypass surgery can affect memory, sometimes transiently and sometimes permanently.
- Chemotherapy can cause sleep difficulty.
- Head trauma, Parkinson's disease, Huntington's disease, multiple sclerosis can also affect sleep.
- Celiac disease is a hereditary disease that occurs in about 1 percent of the population, and is related to a severe reaction to gluten present in wheat, barley, and rye. Fatigue and mental fuzziness are common symptoms.

If you or a loved one are experiencing memory or thinking difficulties, be sure that sleep is adequate, that medications aren't contributing (check with your pharmacist), and that medical conditions aren't a factor.

ALZHEIMER'S

PROTECT YOUR BRAIN FROM ALZHEIMER'S WITH PLANTS, NOT PILLS

This health tip is about preventing Alzheimer's, based on Dr. Neal Barnard's evidence-based book *Power Foods for the Brain*. Other physicians have websites and have written books on this subject, but many of these books are not based on good science, and many of the authors are biased because they sell supplements.

Dr. Barnard is founding president of the respected PCRM (Physician Committee for Responsible Medicine). His book has a chapter about "foods that build your vitamin shield." Vitamin E and three B vitamins—B6, B12, and folic acid—protect against cognitive impairment when ingested in a plant-based diet. However, studies using these vitamins in supplement form indicate they are not beneficial, and can even cause harm:

- Vitamin E pills in doses over 400 units a day increase the risk of heart disease.
- Vitamin A pills in smokers increase the risk of lung cancer.
- Folate is found in many vegetables. Folic acid, present in many vitamin pills and in fortified food is made artificially and is not exactly the same as natural folate. There is evidence that folic acid increases cancer risk.

We evolved to get vitamins, minerals, and other micronutrients through the food we eat. Sudden, huge doses of vitamins in pill or liquid form are not natural, and can cause harm such as oxidation and inflammation that contribute to several maladies including heart disease, cancer, and dementia.

According to Dr. Barnard, here's how you can get brain-healthy vitamins through what you eat:

- Traces of vitamin E are present in broccoli, spinach, sweet potatoes, mangoes, and avocados. Larger amounts are found in nuts and seeds—particularly almonds, walnuts, hazelnuts, pine nuts, pecans, pistachios, sunflower seeds, sesame seeds, and flaxseed. Dr. Barnard mentions a study that showed that "every 5 mg. of vitamin E in a person's diet reduced the risk of developing Alzheimer's disease by 26 percent."
- Best sources of B6 are whole grains, green vegetables, beans, sweet potatoes, bananas, and nuts.

- Sources of folate are broccoli, green leafy vegetables, beans, peas, citrus fruits, and cantaloupe.
- The caveat is that there is one supplement we should take, particularly if we are vegan: vitamin B12, which is made by bacteria in dirt. B12 is found in meat, fortified cereals, fortified soy milk, and nutritional yeast. With treated water and pre-washed produce, most of us don't eat much dirt these days. Vegans should take a 1,000 mg. B12 supplement daily, and Dr. Barnard argues that even meat-eaters should take a daily 2.5 mg. supplement, particularly if over age 50 (older people don't absorb B12 from their diet as well).

While it hasn't been proven that Alzheimer's is a vascular disease yet, we know that Alzheimer's patients have clogged arteries in their brains, and that the risk factors for heart disease (such as hypertension, high cholesterol, smoking, diabetes) are also risk factors for Alzheimer's. Therefore, what's good for the heart is good for the brain. Avoid or at least cut back on meat, dairy, eggs, processed food, added oil, salt, and sugar. Eat mostly—or ideally exclusively—vegetables, fruit, whole grains, nuts, and seeds.

In a video on his website *nutritionfacts.org*, Dr. Michael Greger talked about the marked increase in Alzheimer's in Japan over the past few decades, as meat, dairy, and egg consumption increased by 500 percent. We know what we need to do to ensure healthy brains as we age. Why is it so difficult, then, for so many Americans to modify their lifestyle?

"I don't mind dying so much,
but I don't want it to be my fault."

– Kim Williams, M.D.,
past president of the American College of Cardiology
when asked why he decided to go plant-based.

ALZHEIMER'S

THE IMPORTANCE OF EXERCISE IN PREVENTING ALZHEIMER'S

Neal Barnard, M.D., is the founding president of Physician Committee for Responsible Medicine (PCRM), and one of the giants in nutrition research. He has written several books, including *Power Foods For The Brain, An Effective 3-Step Plan to Protect Your Mind and Strengthen Your Memory.* The 3 steps are diet, exercise, and avoiding common physical threats to brain health such as sleep disruptions and certain medications and medical conditions.

Here are some of the studies that show that physical exercise is important for optimal brain health:

- In a Columbia University study, deconditioned people in the 21 to 45 age range were asked to exercise for 40 minutes, 4 times a week for 12 weeks. Brain MRIs were done before and after the study began. After 12 weeks of exercise, the exercisers' brains had developed new blood vessels and brain cells.

- A University of Illinois study involved 59 sedentary people over age 60. After 6 months of aerobic exercise 3 times a week, their brains were larger than on pre-exercise MRIs.

- The hippocampus is a part of the brain that is important in short and long-term memory, and it typically shrinks by about 1–2 percent per year. In a study, 120 older sedentary adults were asked to start a simple walking program, starting at 10 minutes and working up to 40 minutes 3 times a week. Brain MRIs done before and after showed the hippocampus in these exercisers increased in size. Memory performance also improved.

- A study done by researchers in Seattle's Group Health Cooperative looked at adults over age 65 and found that those who exercised 3 times a week were 40 percent less likely to develop dementia.

- Swedish researchers found that active people were 60 percent less likely to develop Alzheimer's compared to couch potatoes. The positive effect of exercise was particularly evident in those with the ApoE4 gene, a gene that increases the risk of Alzheimer's (an example of how "genetics loads the gun, environment pulls the trigger"—so exercise helps prevent the trigger from being pulled in these people).

According to Dr. Barnard, the explanation for why exercise prevents Alzheimer's is twofold: Exercise plus a healthful diet keeps "your arteries clear and open, maintaining a good blood supply," enabling oxygen to get into the brain and wastes to come out. The second part of the explanation involves brain-derived neurotrophic factor (BDNF), which "helps the brain grow new connections … between brain cells and protects the cells and connections you already have." Aerobic exercise increases brain BDNF.

How much should you exercise? The recommendations are the same as for optimal cardiovascular health. In his book *How Not to Die*, Dr. Greger recommends 90 minutes a day of moderate-intensity exercise (e.g. bicycling on the level, dancing, downhill skiing, hiking, housework, brisk walking) or 40 minutes of vigorous activity (e.g. bicycling uphill, cross-country skiing, jogging, swimming laps). However, huge benefits occur from even mildly-intense exercise, and I tell my patients to exercise aerobically at least 30 minutes a day, hard enough so they can talk but not sing.

"Some people think a plant-based, whole food diet is extreme.
Half a million people a year will have their chests opened up
and a vein taken from their leg and sewn into their coronary artery.
Some people would call that extreme."

– Caldwell Esselstyn, M.D.

ALZHEIMER'S

ANTIBIOTICS, DON'T OVERUSE

There are many organisms that cause harm and even death in humans and animals, including bacteria, viruses, fungi, and parasites. Anti-infective agents have been developed against some but not all organisms in these various classes, but this health tip is about antibiotics, which are active against bacteria.

Prior to the antibiotic era, people in the U.S. died by the thousands every year from infectious diseases such as pneumonia, meningitis, tuberculosis, whooping cough, tetanus, diphtheria, soft tissue infections that spread to the blood stream, and rheumatic fever (a complication of infection by strep bacteria). In 1928, Alexander Fleming found that mold in a petri dish prevented growth of bacteria, and thereby discovered penicillin, which was first produced as a drug in the in the early 1940s. I often hear patients say they don't want to take pharmaceuticals, but antibiotics can clearly be lifesaving. We should feel fortunate to live in an age when many pre-antibiotic-era causes of death and disability can be treated and prevented.

However, it is true that antibiotics do have a downside. First of all, they can have side effects, including severe allergic reactions that can lead to death. Second, in part due to indiscriminate use of antibiotics, bacteria are becoming resistant to antibiotics, which is a huge problem. Eighty percent of antibiotics in this country go to farm animals. Conscientious farmers only use antibiotics for sick animals, but factory farms often use them routinely, to "prevent illness," which leads to antibiotic resistance.

Regarding human use, doctors are criticized for over-prescribing antibiotics, and patients for demanding them. Half of antibiotics prescribed in the U.S. are for viral infections, such as colds and flu, even though viruses do not respond to antibiotics. Admittedly, it's not always easy to differentiate between a viral and a bacterial infection. For example, bacterial pneumonia is usually associated with a high white blood count and a classic white patch on a chest X-ray, but there can be exceptions. The rule of thumb is that if a patient has a high fever, shaking chills, and other signs of severe infection that could possibly be caused by bacteria, they should be covered with antibiotics until blood culture results are back, which could take a day or two.

So, don't go see your doctor for cold symptoms (sore throat, runny nose, aching, mild cough) and demand an antibiotic. It's best to let him or her know that you prefer not to have an antibiotic unless one is truly indicated. The easiest thing for a doctor to do is give you a prescription for an antibiotic and get you out the door, but a conscientious provider will take the time to explain why an antibiotic isn't needed, if indeed it isn't.

A final point is that there are now immunizations against some bacteria. Many immunizations prevent viral diseases, such as polio, measles, German measles, and hepatitis B. But others prevent bacterial infections such as pertussis (whooping cough), tetanus, diphtheria, and pneumococcal infections (the most common cause of pneumonia, among other things). Some patients worry about side effects from immunizations, but they are extremely rare, and the benefit far outweighs any possible risk. Check with your provider, or the CDC website for currently recommended immunizations, and make sure you and your children are up to date.

ANTIBIOTICS

"I know of nothing else in medicine
that can come close to what a plant-based diet can do.
In theory, if everyone were to adopt this,
I really believe we can cut health care costs
by seventy to eighty percent."

– T. Colin Campbell, PhD

ANTIOXIDANTS

DON'T RUST,
EAT ANTIOXIDANT-RICH FOOD

Oxidation involves the removal of electrons from atoms or molecules, creating unstable particles called free radicals. In their book *Beat the Heart Attack Gene,* Bale and Doneen state that oxidative stress is "an imbalance between formation of free radicals and protective antioxidant defenses." An example of oxidation in nature is rusting of metal. Another example is the white of an apple turning brown when you cut it in half and leave it out—the peel doesn't turn brown because that's where most of the antioxidants are. In our bodies, oxidative stress contributes to aging, cancer, and cardiovascular disease.

The following lead to oxidative stress:
- Smoking
- Lack of exercise
- Too much exercise such as running ultra-marathons, repeated marathons, or iron man triathlons
- Unhealthy diet

Antioxidants neutralize oxidative stress, and are found in abundance in fruit and vegetables. Vegetables with intense color such as greens, peppers, red cabbage, red onions, and yams are particularly high in antioxidants. So are intensely-colored fruits such as berries, oranges, and mangoes. Foods with intense flavor such as herbs and spices are also loaded with antioxidants. You can find out how many antioxidants various foods contain by going to *http://bit.ly/antioxidantfoods*. Researchers who put this list together said "antioxidant rich foods originate from the plant kingdom while meat, fish and other foods from the animal kingdom are low in antioxidants." Here are some examples:
- Iceberg lettuce, one of the plant foods with the least nutrients: 17 antioxidant units
- Fresh salmon: 3 units
- Chicken: 5 units
- Skim milk and hard-boiled eggs: 4 units each

- Egg Beaters: 0 units
- Cherries: 714 units
- Some berries have 1,000 units

There is a lab test called F2 isoprostane that Bale and Doneen call the "lifestyle lie detector" because it is a biomarker for oxidative stress. A normal level is less than 0.86, while optimal is less than 0.25. Elevated results occur in people with unhealthy lifestyles and also in over-exercisers.

Supplement and pharmaceutical companies have tried to jump on the antioxidant band wagon and sell antioxidant pills. However, we evolved to get our nutrients by chewing our food, not by taking pills. As Dr. Esselstyn (featured in the *Forks Over Knives* documentary available on YouTube and Netflix, author of *Prevent and Reverse Heart Disease*) says, if we present our body with a "symphony of nutrients" by eating plants, our body has an amazing ability to take out what it needs. If we overwhelm our body with huge doses of single antioxidants and other nutrients in the form of pills, and even juicing and smoothies, this causes problems. For example, the antioxidant vitamins are A, C, and E, but studies show that people who take over 400 units a day of vitamin E in pill form have more heart disease, and smokers who take vitamin A supplements have more lung cancer.

For optimal health, you need lots of antioxidants in your diet and the way to get them is by eating plants—especially by "eating the rainbow"— and chewing your food.

"An educated patient is empowered;
thus, more likely to become healthy."

– Dean Ornish, M.D.

ANTIOXIDANTS

ASPIRIN, TAKE IT OR NOT?

It always amazes me when patients say they don't want to take any medication, but are taking daily aspirin because they heard it might be a good thing to do, without knowing the pros and cons. The answer to whether one should take aspirin is not simple, but here it is:

Aspirin (salicylic acid), in the form of willow bark extract, has been used for thousands of years for pain, fever, and inflammation, and has been available in pill form since 1897. It is also in many fruits and vegetables, with the highest concentration being in herbs and spices, particularly chili powder, paprika, and turmeric. Aspirin from any source acts as an anti-coagulant and helps prevent a blood clot from forming when atherosclerotic plaque ("hardening of the arteries") ruptures, blocking off the blood supply, causing a heart attack or stroke. Aspirin also helps prevent several forms of cancer, particularly colorectal, stomach, and esophageal cancer (less clearly prostate, breast, and lung).

However, just because something is "natural" doesn't mean it can't have side effects. The downside of aspirin is it can cause brain hemorrhage (hemorrhagic stroke), stomach ulcers, and life-threatening stomach bleeding. And some people are allergic to aspirin. If you do take aspirin, you should only take a baby aspirin (81 mg.), because an adult aspirin (325 mg.) is associated with a higher rate of side effects.

There is general agreement among medical experts that if you have had a cardiovascular event (heart attack, atherosclerotic stroke), you should take an 81 mg. aspirin a day to help prevent another event, as long as you don't have a contraindication such as history of an ulcer or stomach bleeding. For the rest of us, organizations such as the U.S. Preventative Task Force, the American Heart Association, and the American Diabetic Association each have their own recommendations, all of which are based on the risk of having a cardiovascular event in the next 10 years. And they keep changing their recommendations, which means they don't really know what's best. If you want to read more about "the party line" on aspirin and heart health, go to *tinyurl.com/aspirinWL*. For more about aspirin and cancer, see *tinyurl.com/aspirinWL2*.

Here's what the experts whom I respect the most say: Brad Bale, M.D., and Amy Doneen, FNP, PhD, in their book *Beat The Heart Attack Gene*, feel the risk score mentioned above is bogus, and I would agree. They want to know what your arteries look like, and to determine that they order a carotid IMT or a coronary calcium score. If you have atherosclerosis, you are at risk for a cardiovascular event and you should take a daily 81 mg. aspirin if you don't have contraindications. If your arteries are clean, the risk outweighs the possible benefit. Furthermore, they point out that 30 percent of Americans have aspirin resistance, meaning 81 mg. of aspirin a day is causing risk but providing no benefit. This can be measured by a simple $20 test, which unfortunately few providers recommend. If you are shown to be aspirin-resistant, you need to be taking a higher dose of aspirin, or possibly another anti-coagulant such as Plavix (some people have resistance to Plavix as well, which can be determined by a genetic test).

Michael Greger, M.D. (*nutritionfacts.org*) looks at this a different way. In his recent book *How Not to Die* (from cardiovascular disease, cancer, etc.) he asks: Wouldn't it be nice if there were a way we all could take daily, low dose aspirin to help prevent cardio-vascular events and cancer, without having the potential side effects? Well there is, but it's in the form of the produce mentioned in the second paragraph, rather than a pill. You might ask why there are no side effects from the salicylic acid in plants, and the an-swer is that "in plants, the salicylic acid appears to come naturally prepackaged with gut-protective nutrients, such as nitric oxide that boosts blood flow and protective mucus production in the lining of the GI tract."

"Seeds and nuts are indispensable
for cardiovascular health."

– Joel Fuhrman, M.D.

ASPIRIN

ATHLETIC PERFORMANCE AND DIET

More elite athletes are embracing plant-based nutrition. A few do it for animal rights or environmental reasons, but most do it for their health and to enhance their performance.

There are three health issues that make elite athletes go plant-based. The first is that when athletes come down with an illness, such as the flu or common cold, they either miss performances or have sub-par performances. Eating plants improves immunity, which helps prevent these illnesses. The second is that athletes such as football linemen are often overweight, which leads to heart disease, diabetes, and early death. All these conditions can be prevented, and diabetes and heart disease can be reversed with plant-based nutrition. The third reason athletes are going plant-based is that intense workouts and athletic performances cause inflammation, tendonitis, and degenerative arthritis. A plant-based diet is anti-inflammatory while a diet based on animal products causes and intensifies inflammation.

Performance enhancement with plant power works like this: Although moderate exercise is good for us, the intense and prolonged exercise that elite athletes engage in causes free radicals and oxidative stress. These in turn lead to aging, inflammation, and slow recovery from workouts. Whole (unprocessed) plants have a multitude of antioxidants (animal products have few to none). Plant-based athletes are able to intensify their workouts, gain strength without gaining fat, recover faster, and lengthen their careers.

What about just taking antioxidant vitamins (A, E, and C), or antioxidant supplements? Theoretically they would help, but studies show they do not and can even be harmful. For example, smokers who take vitamin A supplements have more lung cancer, and people have more heart disease if they take high-dose vitamin E supplements.

Ed Troy is a 60-year-old personal trainer in Colorado, who is an elite masters athlete. He went plant-based a few years ago, dropped some weight, but remained just as strong. He feels better and his performance has improved. The clients who have followed his nutritional advice have noticed the same benefits.

Here is a small sample of elite, vegan athletes:

- Scott Jurek, who is a famous ultra-marathoner, became plant-based as a teenager because he found out that plants have the most nutrients per calorie, important for someone who runs 100-mile races and longer. He wrote an interesting book called *Eat and Run.*

- Carl Lewis, one of the greatest track and field athletes in history, dominated the sprints and long jump during the 1980s and 90s. He was and remains a vegan.

- NFL player David Carter, "the 300 pound vegan," grew up in L.A. on barbecue from his family's restaurant. He developed high blood pressure in his 20s, requiring medication. He also developed tendonitis, arthritis, and nerve damage. He resisted his wife's veganism but went plant-based on February 14, 2014 after watching the documentary *Forks Over Knives.* He says, "The more I learned, the more my body benefited and my results came quickly. More energy, shorter recovery time, increased stamina, improved strength … "

- Tennis star Venus Williams went vegan after being diagnosed with Sjorgren's Disease, an auto-immune disorder that causes joint pain, fatigue, and shortness of breath. Her career suffered and almost ended but was resurrected after she became plant-based.

- MLB pitcher Pat Neshek says, "The main reason I became vegan was the book *The China Study*—it really changed my career."

- Boxer Timothy Bradley says being vegan makes him a better fighter.

- Body builder Torre Washington says, "Vegan athletes are making an international impact on mainstream fitness."

- Body builder Holly Noll says, "Being vegan is not a hindrance but rather a tool to make you the very best you can be."

- UFC fighter Mac Danzig says, "I realized how absurd the notion of 'needing' meat in the diet was. I never looked back … View it as a positive change and look forward to all of the new amazing, healthy, and delicious foods you can eat."

- Ed Bauer, champion bodybuilder says, "Other Bodybuilders eat steak, chicken, eggs, whey protein. I just eat vegan versions of that; tempeh, tofu, seitan, rice and pea protein, some nuts and seeds, spinach and broccoli."

So maybe that "Got Milk?" ad should be changed to "Got Kale?" Unfortunately, there is no "Big Kale" similar to "Big Dairy" to pay for ads like that. Plants have all the protein we need (witness horses, elephants and oxen—"strong as an ox"). Experts such as Dr. Michael Greger (*nutritionfacts.org*) offer proof that plant protein is healthier for us than animal protein.

ATHLETICS

DOPING WITH BEETS

The term "doping" is used with tongue-in-cheek, because this health tip is not about anything illegal or dangerous. According to Michael Greger (*nutritionfacts.org* website, *How Not to Die* book), some five years ago researchers showed that beets and beet juice could improve athletic performance. A drink of beet juice allowed free divers to hold their breath for 30 seconds longer. Cyclists were able to perform at the same level of intensity while consuming 19 percent less oxygen than the placebo group, and when pushing themselves as hard as they could go, the time to exhaustion was extended from 9 min. 43 seconds to 11 min. 15 seconds. Runners who ate 1.5 cups of baked beets 75 minutes before a 5K race improved their performance while maintaining the same heart rate and reporting less exertion. Green leafy vegetables have been shown to do the same thing.

So how does this work? Beets and green leafy vegetables contain nitrates, which the body converts to nitric oxide, which improves the function of the endothelial lining of the arteries, a very delicate but important organ. This in turn causes the arteries to dilate, delivering more blood and oxygen to your heart and other muscles (this is how nitroglycerin works for heart problems, and Viagra for erectile dysfunction). As a result, athletic performance improves. Furthermore, these foods actually enable your body to extract more energy from oxygen, something that researchers previously thought was impossible.

The top ten food sources of nitrates, in descending order of content, are: arugula with the most, then rhubarb, cilantro, butter leaf lettuce, mesclun greens, basil, beet greens, oak leaf lettuce, Swiss chard, and beets. The dose for "doping with plants," based on the plants that have been studied, is 1/2 cup of beet juice or three, 3-inch beets, or a cup of cooked spinach two or three hours before a competition.

LOW BACK PAIN

Low back pain is one of the most common reasons patients see primary care doctors. To understand low back pain, it is necessary to understand the anatomy of the back.

The lumbar (lower back) spine consists of 5 vertebrae, L-1 through L-5, stacked on top of each other. The sacrum and coccyx ("tail bone") are located below L-5. The vertebrae articulate (join) with each other via the facet joints, located in the back of each vertebra. The spinal cord runs through a vertical hole behind the round vertebral bodies. Pads called discs are located between each pair of vertebrae, and serve as cushions—each disc consists of a fibrous band around the outside called the annulus fibrosis, and a soft, jelly-like center. There are nerve fibers in the annulus fibrosis. Nerves to the lower body, including legs, exit between the vertebrae.

Muscles attach to the vertebrae, and the most common back injury is a simple muscle strain, often from lifting improperly, such as twisting while lifting or using your back rather than your legs to lift. Strains are more apt to occur in people who are poorly conditioned and therefore weak, particularly when the supporting core muscles of abdomen are weak. People with a low back strain typically have pain in the area of the strained muscle, made worse with forward, backward, or sideways bending. Treatment is intermittent ice for up to 48 hours, then heat. The safest analgesic is acetaminophen, with aspirin and anti-inflammatories such as ibuprofen or naproxen having more side effects. Symptoms usually resolve within several days. Although people with back strain should avoid activities that cause increased pain, bed rest is counterproductive and "active recovery" such as walking is best. X-rays are not necessary. If the symptoms persist, physical therapy and chiropractic manipulation can be helpful.

Arthritis of the facet joints can cause back pain, and usually occurs in middle-aged or older people. The pain is usually located deep in the back, just to one side of the midline, and often radiates into the buttock. Another cause of back pain is a strain of the S.I. (sacro-iliac) joint— the immovable joint where the pelvic bone joins the tail bone. S.I. strain typically causes pain to one side of the sacrum, often radiating into the thigh. People with this often complain of pain in their "hip."

Another cause of back pain is an injury to a disc, again often caused by improper lifting. A disc can develop a bulge, like a weak spot in a tire or a balloon, and when the

BACK PAIN

annulus fibrosis bulges, the stretched nerve fibers cause pain, usually in the center and to one side of the back. If the bulging disc touches one of the nerve fibers exiting the spinal cord, pain or numbness and tingling can occur down the leg, sometimes to the foot. Disc injuries often heal with time, and again active recovery is best. X-rays are usually not helpful, at least initially, although if symptoms persist, an MRI can help delineate what is going on. If weakness in a leg occurs, by all means seek medical attention—often surgery is indicated. If problems with bowels or bladder occur, that could mean nerves going to these structures are injured, and surgical treatment is urgent.

Back fusions are major operations with long recoveries, and are controversial except in cases of back instability caused by injuries or certain degenerative conditions of the spine. "Failed Back Syndrome" is when a person has had 1 or more operations and their pain is no better or even worse.

Finally, some serious, even life-threatening conditions such as tumors and abdominal aneurysms can cause low back pain. So, if you have significant back pain with no obvious injury, which is not made worse by bending, seek medical attention right away so that a serious condition can be ruled out or treated.

"Food choices are the most significant cause of disease and premature death."

– Joel Fuhrman, M.D.

HOW TO AVOID AND SURVIVE BREAST CANCER

Breast cancer is the most common cancer in American women, after skin cancer. Every year about 230,000 women in this country are diagnosed with breast cancer, and 40,000 die from it. Mammograms and self-breast exams supposedly lead to early detection, but in reality this is "late detection" because breast cancer has been present for years—up to a few decades—by the time it is diagnosed. Some of the 2 billion cells in our bodies are always mutating. We evolved to eat plants, and plants contain micronutrients that destroy these mutant cells before they propagate; animal products lack this ability.

Caldwell Esselstyn, M.D., is one of the two doctors (Dr. Ornish was the other) who proved that plant-based, whole food nutrition with no salt, sugar, or added oil reverses heart disease. Dr. Esselstyn, now in his 80s, started out as a surgeon at the Cleveland Clinic decades ago. He was operating on young women who presented with breast cancer, and the treatment back then was radical mastectomy—a very disfiguring operation. Dr. Esselstyn started looking for a way to prevent breast cancer and found out that breast cancer was rare in plant-based populations.

If you are a woman and want to do everything you can to prevent breast cancer, read the chapter on breast cancer in Dr. Greger's book *How Not to Die*, and search breast cancer on his website *nutritionfacts.org*. If you are a breast cancer survivor, read *The Cancer Survivor's Guide, Foods That Help You Fight Back!* by Neal Barnard, M.D. Following are some of the points made in these two books:

- In 2014 the World Health Organization upgraded its classification of alcohol to "a definitive human breast carcinogen." The culprit is acetaldehyde, a toxic breakdown product of alcohol. Dr. Greger notes that the skin of grapes used to make red wine contains a compound that "may help cancel out some of the cancer-causing effects of the alcohol."
- Melatonin, the "sleep hormone," appears to have a protective effect against breast cancer. Melatonin levels are lowered by bright lights, including computer and TV screens during pre-bedtime hours and by eating meat (for unknown reasons). Eating vegetables raises melatonin levels (again, for unknown reasons).

- Excess estrogen increases breast cancer risk, and women need to be hesitant about taking post-menopausal hormones ("bio-identical hormones" have not been proven to be any safer). Body fat produces estrogen, and therefore people who are overweight are at increased risk for breast cancer.
- Diets high in saturated fat from added oil (coconut oil has the most), meat, dairy products, and eggs increase breast cancer risk.
- Regular exercise such as brisk walking for an hour a day lowers the percentage of body fat, and for that and other reasons, exercise lowers breast cancer risk.
- Heterocyclic amines (HCAs) are carcinogens produced by cooking beef, pork, and other meat—and fish and poultry—at high temperatures, such as roasting, pan frying, grilling, and baking. According to Dr. Greger, "One of the most abundant HCAs in cooked meat, was found to have potent estrogen-like effects, fueling human breast-cancer cell growth."
- Lignans are phytoestrogens that "dampen the effects of the body's own estrogen," according to Dr. Greger. Lignans are particularly plentiful in flaxseeds, and are also found in berries, whole grains, and dark, leafy greens. Flaxseed has even been shown to reduce breast cancer tumor growth. Antibiotics kill health-promoting gut bacteria, which are important in activating lignans.
- According to Dr. Greger, some studies have shown a link between high cholesterol levels and breast cancer risk, thought to be due to our bodies "using cholesterol to make estrogen or to shore up tumor membranes to help the cancer migrate and invade more tissue." Using statins to lower cholesterol does not decrease breast cancer risk.
- Fiber, which is found only in plant foods, helps remove estrogen via the GI tract and lowers breast cancer risk. For every 20 grams of fiber intake per day, there was a 15 percent lower risk of breast cancer in several studies.
- Apple peels contain a compound that activates a breast tumor-suppressor gene.
- Cancerous stem cells may be why breast cancer sometimes recurs years after apparently successful treatment. Sulforaphane, a compound in cruciferous vegetables (e.g. broccoli, cabbage, kale, cauliflower), "suppresses the ability of breast cancer stem cells to form tumors," according to Dr. Greger. Cooking destroys the enzyme that activates sulforaphane, so some cruciferous vegetables should be eaten raw (or eat some raw ones before eating cooked cruciferous vegetables).
- Soybeans contain weak phytoestrogens (phyto = plant) called isoflavones, which attach to estrogen receptors in breast tissue, preventing stronger estro-

gens from attaching, thereby lowering breast cancer risk. It is thought that high soy intake is why the incidence of breast cancer is low in Asian women. If you are a breast cancer survivor, you should know that according to Dr. Greger, "Women diagnosed with breast cancer who ate the most soy lived significantly longer and had a significantly lower risk of breast cancer recurrence."

"The American health care system is like an overflowing sink—
instead of turning off the faucet, providers keep mopping up the floor,
with the hospital and pharmaceutical industries
happily providing the mops and paper towels."

– Original author unknown

CANCER

HOW TO PREVENT AND SURVIVE PROSTATE CANCER

The prostate is a gland that is the size and shape of a walnut, and surrounds the urethra (the outlet of the bladder). Prostate cancer is the second most common cancer in American men, after skin cancer. A 50-year-old American man has a 40 percent risk of eventually developing slow-growing, non-fatal prostate cancer that will never cause symptoms or kill him; a 16 percent risk of developing prostate cancer that will cause symptoms and require some type of treatment; and a 2.9 percent risk of fatal prostate cancer.

PSA (prostate specific antigen) is a blood test used to detect prostate cancer, although conditions such as prostate infection can also elevate it. PSA is not a perfect test because elevation does not differentiate between slow-growing and more aggressive, deadly cancer. If aggressive cancer is identified, radical prostatectomy can be life-saving, but often results in side effects such as impotence and bladder leakage. Side effects are also common with chemotherapy and radiation.

Prevention of prostate cancer is the best approach. Some men have a genetic predisposition for prostate cancer, but as is often the case, what you eat determines whether or not these genes will be turned on. Some of the 2 billion cells in our bodies are always mutating. Plants contain micronutrients that kill off these abnormal cells before they multiply and end up as cancer; animal products don't have nutrients that do that. Dr. Dean Ornish proved over 25 years ago that a plant-based, whole food diet with no salt, sugar, or added oil reverses heart disease. In his book *The Spectrum*, he discusses a more recent study in which he proved this diet can reverse early prostate cancer and can slow the progression of aggressive, metastatic prostate cancer. Here is how you can prevent prostate cancer, and if you already have it how you can reverse or slow the progression of it:

- Avoid cows' milk, which is good for baby cows but is problematic for humans of any age. In his book *How Not to Die*, Dr. Michael Greger notes that "nutrition experts have expressed concern that the hormones in dairy products and other growth factors could stimulate the growth of hormone-sensitive tumors," including prostate cancer. One of these growth factors is IGF-1 (insulin growth factor-1), which makes baby cows grow rapidly but which in adult humans stimulates the growth of cancer cells.

- Avoid eggs. Dr. Greger presents evidence that choline in eggs is converted into a toxin called trimethylamine by our gut bacteria, which when oxidized by the liver increases the risk of prostate cancer. Eating even a few eggs a week doubles the risk of prostate cancer progression such as bone metastases.
- Avoid cooked meat, including red meat and poultry. Cooking meat causes carcinogens such as heterocyclic amines (HCAs) to form.
- Avoid fatty foods because they increase the risk of prostate cancer.
- Increase your intake of fruit and vegetables because they decrease prostate cancer risk by killing off mutant cells as soon as they form. According to Dr. Neal Barnard in *The Cancer Survivor's Guide,* plant-based foods also cause a "drop in the biochemical factors such as hormones that stimulate (prostate) cancer growth."
- Be wary of taking testosterone supplements because they can stimulate growth of prostate cancer.

The bottom line, according to Dr. Barnard, is that "by boosting vegetables, fruits, beans, and whole grains, and avoiding dairy products, meats, eggs, and fried foods, men are able to take advantage of protective nutrients and avoid cancer-promoting factors." Up through World War 2, prostate cancer was very rare in Japan. Sadly, the rate of prostate cancer there has increased significantly since then, as the Japanese diet has become more Westernized.

"Stop eating when you're 80 percent full."

– Okinawan proverb

HOW TO PREVENT AND SURVIVE COLORECTAL CANCER

About 50,000 Americans die every year from colorectal cancer, but in some parts of the world it's extremely rare. The lining of the colon, with its bumps and crevasses, has a large surface area that comes in contact with the food we eat. It's not surprising, then, that what we eat has a strong influence on our risk for colon cancer.

The earliest stage of colon cancer is clusters of abnormal cells lining the colon. The second stage is polyps—small growths that protrude from the lining. The final stage occurs when small polyps, that are initially benign, slowly become malignant. Eventually, colon cancer extends through the wall of the colon and spreads (metastasizes) through-out the body. Early detection methods such as colonoscopy should be discussed with your primary provider before you turn 50 (some authorities are now saying 45), or earlier if you have a family history of polyps or colon cancer.

What a lot of people, including many health-care providers, don't know is that for the most part, colon cancer can be prevented.* Following are some suggestions from Dr. Michael Greger's book *How Not to Die* and his website *nutritionfacts.org*. Another good source of information is *The Cancer Survivor's Guide* by Neal Barnard, M.D.

- Eat 1/4 to 1/2 teaspoonfuls of turmeric a day, available in bulk at Vitamin Cottage. Turmeric in curry is thought to contribute to the low rate of colon cancer in India. When turmeric is added to cancer cells in the lab, they stop multiplying. When turmeric comes in contact with the lining of the colon, it prevents abnormal cells from forming, and if abnormal cells are already present, they revert to normal. Familial polyposis is a genetic disease in which family members develop multiple colon polyps, often resulting in colon cancer. When people with this condition are given daily turmeric, the number and size of polyps decreases by half. Even advanced colon cancer resistant to chemotherapy and radiation regressed with oral or rectal (via enema) turmeric in one study. Curcumin, a component of turmeric available in supplement form, is not as effective as unprocessed turmeric.
- Eat foods containing quercetin, another plant nutrient that has been shown to decrease colon polyps and risk for colon cancer. Quercetin is found in such

fruits and vegetables as grapes and red onions.

- Eat foods that contain phytates—another cancer-preventing plant nutrient, found in green, leafy vegetables; legumes (beans, split peas, chickpeas and lentils); whole grains; and nuts and seeds.
- Eat high-fiber food. Fiber, which is present in plant but not animal products, helps prevent colon cancer, in part due to decreasing stool transit time—the time it takes for food to go through the intestinal tract. For example, food goes through men eating plant-based diets in a day or two, but takes 5 or more days in men eating a conventional diet.
- Avoid meat, including poultry and seafood, because they increase the risk of colon cancer, partly because these foods contain heme iron (plants contain non-heme iron). Heme iron causes free radicals that contribute to inflammation and cancer. A six-year study of 30,000 people in California showed the risk of colon cancer doubled in those who ate red meat at least once a week and tripled in those who ate chicken or fish at least once a week.
- "Eat the rainbow," because foods with intense color are loaded with antioxidants, which help prevent many health problems, including cancer. Daily intake of black raspberries for 9 months reduced the number of polyps by half in patients with familial colon polyps.

You'd think that nutritional information like this would be taught in medical schools, but it wasn't when I attended the University of Colorado School of Medicine in the 1960s. I was at my fiftieth medical school reunion in Denver recently and talked to several students from the class of 2018, and things hadn't changed. I'm happy to say though, that at the time this book is going to press, plans are being made to teach medical students in Colorado about nutrition and prevention, starting in 2019-20.

CANCER

HOW TO AVOID CANCER
OF THE ESOPHAGUS

The esophagus is the tube that carries food from your mouth to your stomach. There are about 18,000 new cases of esophageal cancer diagnosed in the U.S. annually, resulting in around 15,000 deaths. Cancer usually starts in the lining of the esophagus, and symptoms are often absent in this stage. Eventually the cancer invades the outer layers of the esophagus, and the final stage involves spread to other organs (metastases).

The primary risk factors for esophageal cancer are smoking, heavy alcohol consumption, and GERD (gastroesophageal reflux disease—acid reflux). According to Dr. Greger in his book *How Not to Die*, over the past 30 years, "the incidence of esophageal cancer in Americans has increased six-fold," primarily due to an increase in GERD. It's interesting that 28 percent of Americans suffer from acid reflux at least weekly, whereas in Asia only 5 percent of the population are affected. The difference is not genetic, because when Asians move here and eat the S.A.D. (Standard American Diet) they suffer the same rate of GERD as the rest of us. The difference is in what they eat in their native countries.

According to Dr. Greger, "The most consistent association with (esophageal cancer) was the consumption of meat and high-fat meals." A few minutes after eating a fatty meal, the sphincter muscle between the lower end of the esophagus and the stomach relaxes, allowing acid to backflow into the esophagus, where is doesn't belong, which causes a burning sensation in the chest (heartburn). Over the years, the chronic irritation and inflammation from acid reflux leads to Barrett's esophagus, which is a pre-cancerous abnormality of the lower esophagus. Eventually, cancer often ensues. (Scarring of the lower esophagus can also occur, which results in difficulty swallowing food.)

Fiber, which is found in plant but not animal products, decreases reflux and reduces the risk of esophageal cancer by at least one-third. Fiber prevents constipation and straining at the stool, which can cause a hiatal hernia, where part of the stomach is pushed up through the diaphragm, which separates the chest and the abdominal cavities. Hiatal hernias are often the cause of cancer-causing acid reflux. Fiber also binds to and "flushes out" cancer-causing environmental toxins.

Plants not only contain fiber, but they also contain antioxidants and other cancer-killing micronutrients. Dr. Greger notes that "the most protective foods for esophageal cancer are red, orange, and dark-green leafy vegetables, berries, apples, and citrus fruits." In a randomized study, patients with mild to moderate precancerous esophageal lesions were given large quantities of powdered strawberries daily for 6 months, and progression of disease was reversed in 80 percent; in 50 percent the disease totally resolved.

The prognosis of esophageal cancer is grim, with a 5-year survival of less than 20 percent. The tips noted above can help prevent it. But if you have difficulty swallowing, or more than occasional heartburn, see your primary care provider or a gastroenterologist without delay. An upper endoscopy can detect precancerous Barrett's. Acid reducers such as Prilosec and Nexium can help, but when taken long-term can have side effects. I have seen countless patients over the years whose GERD resolved with lifestyle modification such as healthier eating; avoiding aspirin, ibuprofen and other irritating anti-inflammatories; raising the head of the bed; avoiding alcohol and caffeine; and avoiding eating within 2 hours of reclining.

*"People feel poorly because they are nourished
by foods you wouldn't feed to your dog and cat.
The rich Western diet is full of fat, sugar, cholesterol, salt, animal protein
—all the wrong foods for people."*

– John A. McDougall, M.D.

CANCER

HOW TO PREVENT CANCER
OF THE PANCREAS

The pancreas is a large gland located behind the stomach. It secretes insulin, necessary for blood sugar control, directly into the blood stream. It also secretes digestive juices into the small intestine that are necessary for digestion of proteins. About 46,000 Americans develop pancreatic cancer every year, which is impossible to screen for, and is difficult to diagnose early and to treat successfully—few patients diagnosed with pancreatic cancer survive more than a year. Therefore, it's particularly important to prevent this cancer.

Here's how you can stack the deck in your favor to avoid pancreatic cancer, according to Dr. Michael Greger in his book *How Not to Die* and on his website *nutritionfacts.org*:

- Don't smoke—about 20 percent of cases of pancreatic cancer are related to smoking.
- Maintain your ideal body weight because obesity is a risk factor for pancreatic cancer. Check your height and your weight and google your BMI to find out if you're overweight.
- Avoid heavy drinking, which is another risk factor for pancreatic cancer. More than 1 drink a day for women and 2 drinks a day for men is considered unhealthy (note that any alcohol except perhaps a little red wine is a risk factor for breast cancer in women). One drink is defined as 4 ounces of wine, 12 oz beer, or 1 oz of hard alcohol.
- Avoid fat from animal products. Dr. Greger notes that older studies have been conflicting but that the large NIH-AARP study showed that "the consumption of fat from all animal sources was significantly associated with pancreatic cancer risk, but no correlation was found with consumption of plant fats." This means you should avoid meat, including chicken, seafood, eggs, and all dairy products including cheese and yogurt. Instead, get the fat you need in your diet from nuts, seeds (sunflower, pumpkin, flax, chia, hemp), olives, and avocados.
- If you want to avoid pancreatic cancer, it's particularly important that you avoid chicken. In a study of 30,000 poultry workers, their risk of pancreatic cancer

was found to be 9 times the risk in the general population. This is thought to be due to cancer-causing poultry viruses that can be transmitted to humans. Regarding people who eat chicken, a large European study found a 72 percent increase in pancreatic cancer for every 50 grams of chicken eaten daily (50 grams is about 1/4 of a chicken breast).

- Eat 1/4 to 1/2 teaspoonfuls of turmeric a day, which in the lab has been shown to reverse early cancerous changes in pancreatic cells. Larger doses of turmeric taken daily have been shown to be as effective as chemotherapy in delaying progression of pancreatic cancer.

- Avoid foods with a high glycemic index. In his book *Fast Food Genocide,* Dr. Joel Fuhrman notes that these foods are linked to several cancers, including pancreatic. These are foods such as sugary or refined foods that raise your blood sugar rapidly.

- Avoid processed meat (such as sausage, lunch meat, bacon, ham), and fast food. Dr. Fuhrman notes that "increased consumption of processed meat, and meats cooked with typical fast food cooking techniques, correlates positively with the likelihood of developing … pancreatic … cancer." Carcinogens such as heterocyclic amines are formed when muscle meat "including beef, pork, fish, and poultry" is cooked at high temperatures, such as pan frying and grilling.

- Eat cruciferous vegetables daily such as broccoli, cauliflower, kale, cabbage, bok choy, and brussels sprouts. Dr. Fuhrman cites a study showing that one or more servings of cabbage a week reduced risk of pancreatic cancer by 38 percent.

"Tanned skin is not healthy skin."

– Center for Disease Control

CANCER

HOW TO AVOID BLOOD CANCERS

There are basically 3 types of blood cancers: leukemia, lymphoma, and myeloma.

- Leukemia involves propagation of mutant white blood cells in the bone marrow. Normal white blood cells fight infection but leukemia cells lose this function. Furthermore, they crowd out normal red and other types of white blood cells in the bone marrow. Around 52,000 cases of leukemia occur in the U.S. annually, resulting in 24,000 deaths.

- Lymphoma involves mutation and propagation of another type of white blood cell: lymphocytes. The most common type is non-Hodgkin's lymphoma, of which there are 70,000 cases diagnosed in the U.S. every year, with about 19,000 deaths.

- Myeloma involves plasma cells—white blood cells that produce antibodies. Some 24,000 Americans are diagnosed with myeloma every year, resulting in 11,000 deaths.

Treatment of blood cancers has variable results, with the greatest success being childhood leukemia, which now has a 90 percent 10-year survival rate. As with other diseases, prevention is best. In his book *How Not to Die*, Dr. Michael Greger reviews foods associated with decreased blood cancer risk. As discussed in the last several health tips, what we eat and don't eat can lower the risk of many types of cancer. Dr. Greger says studies have shown that "the greatest protection appeared to be against blood cancers."

- Sulforaphane* is a strong cancer-fighting micronutrient present in cruciferous vegetables: arugula, bok choy, broccoli, brussels sprouts, cabbage, cauliflower, collard greens, horseradish, kale, mustard greens, radishes, turnip greens, and watercress. Sulforaphane kills human leukemia cells in the lab, and studies have shown that high daily cruciferous intake decreases the risk of lymphoma.

- In a Mayo Clinic study, people who ate 5 or more servings of green, leafy vegetables a week had 50 percent less lymphoma compared with those eating less than 1 serving a week.

- There is preliminary evidence that turmeric can slow or stop pre-myeloma changes in humans.
- Acai berries have been shown in the lab to be effective against leukemia cells. Studies have not been done yet that show whether they are effective in preventing leukemia in people however. Of course, Big Food jumped on the favorable lab evidence; beware of "superfood" supplements and shakes, which have not been proven to do anything.

Dr. Greger also cites certain foods that increase the risk of blood cancers:
- Growing up around or working around poultry are risk factors for blood cancers. Eating poultry regularly also increases risk. The cause is thought to be certain poultry viruses, which can cause cancer in poultry and probably in humans (we don't know for sure yet).
- "Exposure to cattle and pigs has also been associated with non-Hodgkin's lymphoma, and eating them may prove to increase risk of lymphoma although again, we don't know for sure yet."

In order for sulforaphane to be released, an enzyme called myrosinase is necessary, and this enzyme is inactivated by cooking. If you want to cook some of your cruciferous vegetables, one thing you can do is eat some raw cruciferous veggies such as cauliflower or broccoli before you eat cooked ones—that way myrosinase is available to release sulforaphane. A second strategy is to chop or blend cruciferous veggies at least 40 minutes before you cook them, which allows myrosinase to do its job. A third strategy is to add mustard or horseradish to cooked cruciferous veggies (mustard greens and seeds are cruciferous). Dr. Greger notes that "commercially produced frozen broccoli lacks the ability to form sulforaphane because vegetables are blanched (flash-cooked) before they're frozen" to prolong shelf life.

CANCER

SKIN CANCER –
HOW TO KEEP YOUR SKIN HEALTHY

Many people are in denial about what their arteries look like, but it's hard to be in denial about what your skin looks like. Americans spend billions of dollars every year on anti-aging skin products. Botox injections and cosmetic plastic surgery account for billions more. However, aging of our skin is not caused by deficiency of anti-aging skin creams. This health tip will discuss some factors you need to be aware of if you want to have healthy, young-looking skin:

First of all, don't smoke. Nicotine and other chemicals in cigarettes damage the blood supply to your skin (as well as other parts of your body). They also damage collagen and elastin in your skin, making it saggy.

Second, according to Dr. Michael Greger's website *nutritionfacts.org*, alcohol, especially in large quantities, contributes to skin aging. This is because breakdown products of alcohol decrease carotenoid antioxidants in the skin, which lowers the threshold for sunburn and increases the risk of skin cancer.

Third, ultraviolet radiation from the sun and tanning booths leads to premature aging, including wrinkling; sagging; and pigmented areas called sun, age or liver spots. UV exposure also contributes to pre-cancerous rough, red spots called actinic keratoses; basal cell cancer; squamous cell cancer; and to the often-deadly skin cancer melanoma. We all like being out in the sun, but we should cover up with long-sleeved sun-protective clothing and a broad-brimmed hat. Apply a broad-spectrum (protects against both UVA and UVB rays), high SPF sunscreen to the parts of your body you can't cover up, such as the back of your hands and your lower face. The safest and best sunscreens contain zinc oxide or titanium, which physically block the sun versus sunscreens with chemicals that can be absorbed and could possibly cause harm. Remember, suntanned skin is sun-damaged skin. In Japan, where light, unblotched skin is prized, women wear gloves and use umbrellas when they're out in the sun, and as they age they maintain youthful-looking skin.

Fourth, what you eat affects your skin. Free radicals and oxidation contribute to skin aging and skin cancer. Therefore, it is important to eat food with lots of antioxidants and other cancer-fighting plant micronutrients found in unprocessed plant foods, including vegetables, legumes, fruit, and whole grains. Studies have shown that people who are plant-based are protected from sun damage compared to people who eat mainly animal products. Their immune system is optimal, skin aging slows, and they are at lower risk for actinic keratoses and skin cancer, including melanoma. And plant-based nutrition has been shown to reverse early skin cancer, including melanoma in some cases.

Acne seems to be a disease associated with Western diet, according to experts such as Dr. Greger and Dr. Fuhrman. For example, acne is essentially non-existent in Okinawa and other plant-based parts of the world. In the U.S. some 85 percent of teenagers are afflicted with acne, which often persists into their third decade. Recent studies show a clear correlation between acne and dairy products. A large percentage of milk comes from pregnant cows, and the link with acne appears to be due to hormones in cows' milk. Skim milk is the worst because it has the highest estrogen content. The most antioxidant-packed fruit are dried barberries, which can be found in Middle Eastern markets. One teaspoon 3 times a day for a month resulted in a 43 percent decrease in acne in one study.

Many products marketed as anti-aging are of questionable benefit. However, antioxidant products such as L'dara, applied regularly to the skin, can reduce precancerous actinic keratoses and other signs of skin aging. But it's best to also get your skin antioxidants from the inside out by eating antioxidant-containing food. There is a good plant-based cookbook called *Oh She Glows,* which refers to glowing from the inside out. Healthy, "glowing" skin has a slightly pinkish and yellowish hue, which means it has an abundance of carotenoid antioxidants.

"Nutritional excellence is
the only real fountain of youth."

– Joel Fuhrman, M.D.

CANCER

ATHEROSCLEROSIS (HARDENING OF THE ARTERIES), PART 1

Atherosclerosis is also known as plaque, or hardening of the arteries and is common in Americans and other people on a Western diet as they age. However, it's not normal; it doesn't occur in people who are on a lifelong plant-based, whole food diet with avoidance of salt, sugar, and added oil. These people have blood pressures that don't rise as they get older, have total cholesterols of less than 150, and LDL (bad cholesterol) levels in the 30s and 40s.

Oxygen-poor blood returning to the heart through veins is pumped by the right ventricle of the heart through the lungs, where it takes on oxygen. The left ventricle then pumps blood through arteries to our organs and tissues, including our heart muscle (myocardium). The inside of our arteries is lined by an organ system called the endothelium. If our endothelium is stressed, through bad genes; through bad habits such as smoking, lack of exercise or unhealthy diet; or by conditions such as inflammation, high blood pressure, diabetes or high cholesterol, the endothelium starts to thicken. Eventually, plaque develops.

Ninety-nine percent of plaque is located in the walls of our arteries, causing a blockage. If plaque in a coronary (heart) artery ruptures, a blood clot forms, blocking the blood supply to part of the heart muscle, resulting in a heart attack—the number one cause of death in America. If this happens in an artery in the brain, a stroke occurs—the number one cause of disability in the U.S. and a common cause of death.

Sometimes plaque grows slowly, causing an incomplete obstruction in an artery. If this occurs in a coronary artery, blood flow to the part of the myocardium supplied by that artery is insufficient when the person exerts, such as walking rapidly or walking uphill. This results in angina—chest pain with exertion. When similar blockages occur in the legs, it is called peripheral vascular disease, which causes leg pain if the person walks very far, a condition called claudication. If the blockage becomes severe enough, gangrene of the toes and feet can occur.

Following are some other problems that can occur with incomplete, chronic arterial blockages:

- Plaque in the arteries of the brain contributes to dementia, including Alzheimer's.
- Plaque in the arteries that supply blood to the eyes can lead to loss of vision.
- Plaque in the carotid arteries in the neck behaves somewhat differently than plaque elsewhere, in that small pieces can break off and go to the brain, causing small strokes, or causing TIAs (transient ischemia attacks) that are warning signs of an impending stroke.
- Plaque on heart valves causes narrowing and/or leaking of the valves.
- Plaque in the arteries that supply blood to the intestines can cause "intestinal angina"—abdominal pain after eating. If the blockages become severe enough, intestinal gangrene can occur, necessitating removal of the dead bowel.
- Plaque in the thread-like arteries to the penis leads to erectile dysfunction. E.D. is the "canary in the coal mine," indicating atherosclerosis elsewhere in the body.
- Plaque in arteries to the kidneys can lead to severe high blood pressure and plaque in arteries within the kidneys leads to chronic kidney failure.

"It takes more than a try to quit addictions; it takes a commitment."

– Joel Fuhrman, M.D.

ATHEROSCLEROSIS (HARDENING OF THE ARTERIES), PART 2

Essentially everyone on the S.A.D. (Standard American Diet) has at least some degree of hardening of the arteries, also known as atherosclerosis, or plaque. This is primarily because this diet is high in meat, dairy, eggs, refined food, salt, sugar, and vegetable oil; and low in fruit, vegetables, and whole grains.

Calcified plaque can show up on imaging studies ordered for other reasons; for example, plaque seen in abdominal arteries on X-rays ordered to evaluate back pain, or plaque in the carotid arteries of the neck seen on routine dental X-rays. Heart attack prevention doctors believe it's important to assess their patients' arteries, and to do this they often order carotid IMTs—ultrasound studies of the carotid arteries that pick up early signs of atherosclerosis. Coronary calcium scores—CAT scans of the heart—can also be used to assess arterial health, although false negatives can occur in women under 50 and men under 40, whose plaque has not yet become calcified.

People on a lifelong plant-based, whole (unprocessed) food diet with no salt, sugar, or added oil don't get atherosclerosis. If you aren't on this diet and already have this disease, Dr. Dean Ornish showed over 25 years ago that a plant-based diet plus regular exercise can reverse it, and Dr. Caldwell Esselstyn proved the same thing more recently. Just eating more fruits, vegetables, and whole greens and less meat, dairy, eggs, salt, sugar, and oil helps, but not as much as being 100 percent compliant.

Other measures that help stabilize plaque so that it doesn't cause problems such as heart attacks, and so more doesn't form, are the following:
- Don't smoke.
- Maintain a blood pressure of less than 120/80.
- Maintain ideal body weight, and in particular get rid of your "belly" if you have one. Measure your waist at the point of biggest circumference—approximately at the level of your navel—and if you're a woman the measurement should be less than 35 inches, and if you're a man less than 40 inches (cutoff points are less in Asians and East Indians). If you have belly fat, you undoubtedly have insulin resistance/pre-diabetes.

- Engage in at least 30 minutes of daily aerobic exercise such as brisk walking (at 4 miles per hour).
- Control your lipids. Guidelines are total cholesterol < 200; HDL (good cholesterol) > 40 in a male or postmenopausal female and > 50 in a premenopausal female; triglycerides < 150, LDL (bad cholesterol) < 100 or if you've had a heart attack < 70. However, heart attack-proof levels are: total cholesterol < 150; LDL in the 30s or 40s, triglycerides < 70.
- Diagnose pre-diabetes early, while it's still reversible, by a 2-hour glucose tolerance test (normal is 1-hour < 125 and 2-hour < 120). Ideally reverse it through diet and exercise, although certain medications can be helpful.
- If you have type 2 diabetes, you can reverse it through diet and exercise unless you've had it for a long time. If you don't or can't reverse it, keep your blood sugars and A1C at goal with medication.
- Diagnose and treat sleep apnea.
- Diagnose and treat inflammation, including gum and tooth disease.
- There is a strong mouth-vascular connection, so practice good dental hygiene and see your dentist regularly.
- Get 7–8 hours of good sleep a night.
- Avoid stress; consider mindful meditation.

For people unable or unwilling to get their lipids to goal by diet and exercise, consider a statin drug. Most people tolerate statins well. A minority of patients complain of muscle aching and/or weakness. Heart attack prevention doctors know tricks that help people avoid side effects, and there are also medication alternatives to statins.

"No chemical carcinogen is nearly so important in causing human cancer as animal protein."

– T. Colin Campbell, PhD

WOMEN AND HEART DISEASE

Here's an all-too-common true story, from the book *Beat the Heart Attack Gene* by Brad Bale, M.D. and Amy Doneen, RN, PhD: A 37-year-old woman, J.T., was rushing around getting ready for work in the morning and experienced a sharp pain in her chest, radiating down her right arm, accompanied by shortness of breath. She had no obvious risk factors for heart disease and it didn't occur to her that she might be having a heart attack. She then developed nausea and collapsed on the floor. Her husband drove her to the ER, and after a long wait an EKG was done, which was normal. She was told that because she was a woman and was young, because her pain radiated down her right instead of her left arm, and because her EKG was normal, she wasn't having a heart attack. She was diagnosed with anxiety and bacterial pneumonia and was given azithromycin, an antibiotic that has been shown to triple cardiovascular mortality.

She continued to have symptoms during the night, and the next morning her husband drove her to an urgent care center. The doctor there was skeptical of the pneumonia diagnosis and ordered a blood test for cardiac enzymes, which were very elevated, indicating damage to the myocardium (heart muscle). He wanted to call an ambulance but J.T. was concerned about the cost, so her husband drove her to the ER, where she waited for 2 hours before she was evaluated. Another EKG was normal, but her cardiac enzymes were sky high. Finally, a heart attack was diagnosed and appropriate treatment was started. She was fortunate she lived through this saga, given that in some 20 percent of heart attacks the first symptom is the last: sudden death.

Here's what you need to know about women and heart disease:
- From ages 35 to 85, cancer is the number one killer in women, with heart disease number three from ages 35 to 44, and number two from 45 to 85 after which heart disease is number one.
- Women tend to develop heart disease a decade later than men, but as with men, heart disease is the number one killer in women overall.
- Of the 435,000 American women who have heart attacks every year, 83,000 are under the age of 65, and 35,000 are under 55.
- In men and women, the process that results in heart disease is the same: Damage over the years to the endothelial lining of the arteries, which eventually re-

sults in plaque (hardening of the arteries). In men, heart disease usually affects the larger coronary (heart) arteries, whereas in women smaller arteries are often involved (called microvascular disease).

- In men, classic heart attack symptoms are crushing chest pain often radiating to the jaw or left arm, shortness of breath, nausea, light-headedness, and sweating. Women often have more subtle symptoms, including mild pain in the upper back, shoulders, neck, or either arm; anxiety, and unusual fatigue.
- The American Heart Association says that coronary heart disease in women "remains understudied, underdiagnosed and undertreated." This is especially true of younger women and black women.
- In 20 percent of heart attacks in both women and men, the first symptom of heart disease is the last: sudden death.

How do you know if you have heart disease and are therefore at risk for a heart attack (or stroke)?

- Risk factors in men and women are similar: Smoking; family history; high blood pressure (greater than 120/80); high cholesterol or triglycerides; low HDL (good cholesterol—should be over 50 in premenopausal women and over 40 in postmenopausal); diabetes and pre-diabetes; obesity; lack of exercise; inflammation including dental problems; stress, including depression and anxiety; sleep problems, including sleep apnea.
- Heart attack prevention doctors will want to check the health of your arteries. Bale and Doneen recommend a carotid IMT for this: a non-invasive ultrasound picture of the carotid arteries in the neck, which involves no radiation. Another helpful test is a coronary calcium score, available at most imaging centers and hospitals, but this can be falsely negative in women under age 50 or men under 40 because their plaque hasn't become calcified yet.
- Dr. Caldwell Esselstyn (*Forks Over Knives* documentary, *Prevent and Reverse Heart Disease* book) says anyone on the S.A.D. (Standard American Diet) can be assumed to have heart disease.

In summary, cardiovascular disease is the major cause of death in women, and a major cause of disability (strokes, heart failure). Here's the good news though: Heart disease can be prevented and even reversed with lifestyle modification, consisting of regular exercise and plant-based, whole (unprocessed) food diet with no salt, sugar, or added oil. If you aren't willing to make these lifestyle changes, medications such as statin drugs can be helpful, and some people need medications even if they have an optimal lifestyle (e.g. people with severe atherosclerosis or a familial hyperlipidemia with extreme cholesterol elevation).

CARDIOVASCULAR DISEASE

HOW TO PREVENT A HEART ATTACK

Almost all heart attacks can be prevented but unfortunately many aren't, resulting in unnecessary death and disability. Michael Greger, M.D., has the website *nutrition-facts.org* and wrote *How Not to Die* and he likens our health care system to an over-flowing sink, where instead of turning off the faucet (preventing the cause of disease), we spend our time, effort, and a lot of money constantly mopping up the floor, with the pharmaceutical, hospital, stent and bypass industries happily supplying the mops and the paper towels—at a large profit.

People who exercise regularly and who are on a life-long plant-based diet with no salt, sugar, or added oil, don't develop atherosclerosis and therefore are not at risk for a heart attack. (Unless they have familial hyperlipidemia genetic disease.)

If you have not been on this diet and/or have not been exercising, and don't know if you have plaque (atherosclerosis), you should consider a carotid IMT—an inexpensive, non-invasive test (not the carotid doppler done at hospitals, which is much less sensitive). The IMT study determines the health of the carotid arteries in your neck, and there is a 95 percent correlation with the coronary arteries (heart) arteries. Another option is a coronary calcium score, although false negatives can occur if you are a man under age 40 or a woman under 50 due to plaque that hasn't become calcified yet. If you find that you do have atherosclerosis, you are at risk for a heart attack (and stroke) and here's what you need to do to prevent one:

- Find a primary care doctor who has expertise in heart attack prevention, who will look at your atherosclerosis as a medical disease that can be treated medically rather than a plumbing problem that needs to be treated with stents or bypass which have never been shown to prolong life or improve quality of life other than in the setting of an acute heart attack.
- Find a provider who will help you start a plant-based diet and exercise program, which have been shown to stabilize and even reverse atherosclerosis.
- Don't smoke.
- If you carry extra weight around your middle, or if you have elevated triglycerides and/or low HDL (good cholesterol), insist on a 2-hour glucose tolerance test. If the 1 hour blood sugar is > 125 or the 2 hour >120, you have insulin re-

sistance/pre-diabetes: a condition that is the driver of 70 percent of cardiovascular disease. If caught early, pre-diabetes and even type 2 diabetes are reversible.

- Make sure your blood pressure is less than 120/80 (somewhat higher values may be appropriate if you are elderly and frail).
- Make sure your total cholesterol is less than 150 and your LDL (bad cholesterol) less than 70, with 30s to 40s being ideal.
- Especially if you don't follow the above lifestyle modifications, a statin can help lower your LDL (bad cholesterol) and also decrease inflammation.
- Obtain a Cleveland Heart Lab inflammatory panel, because inflammation plays an important role in causing atherosclerosis, and in plaque rupture—the event that causes heart attacks. Elevated MPO or LpPLA2 means inflammation of the endothelial lining of your arteries and/or plaque and needs to be treated aggressively.
- Have an advanced lipid panel done, including an LDL particle number (Apo B is an equivalent test), which is much more accurate than the LDL level, and which checks for particle size, with small LDL particle size being more worrisome. Lp(a)—a particularly harmful type of LDL particle— should also be included because Lp(a) is responsible for a lot of heart disease.
- Take an 81 mg. aspirin a day, which will help prevent a blood clot from forming should you have plaque that ruptures. Ask your doctor about doing an aspirin resistance test to be sure 81 mg. is enough.
- Consider taking ramipril, a medication usually used to treat blood pressure, that has been shown to stabilize plaque.
- Mouth and gum disease have a huge impact on vascular health. See your dentist immediately if you have dental issues and practice good dental hygiene— brush after meals, floss and use a water pick every night. See your dentist for regular cleaning and on an urgent basis if you have any acute or chronic dental issues.
- If you snore, get checked for sleep apnea, and have it treated if you do have it (just losing weight and avoiding alcohol often helps).
- Get 7–8 hours of sleep at night.
- Consider a class in meditation or mindfulness to reduce stress, anxiety, and depression.
- Read *Beat the Heart Attack Gene* by Brad Bale, M.D. and Amy Doneen, N.P., PhD.
- Read *Prevent and Reverse Heart Disease* by Caldwell Esselstyn, M.D. Keep in mind that he is trying to reverse severe heart disease and that his advice to avoid nuts and seeds is too hard-core for most people, who need those things for brain health.

CARDIOVASCULAR DISEASE

- Have your carotid IMT repeated in a year, to assess effectiveness of your treatment (coronary calcium scores should not be repeated because if soft plaque becomes calcified—which is a good thing because calcified plaque is more stable—the score will be higher).
- If you have chest pain or tightness, have it evaluated immediately.

"To prevent heart attacks it is necessary to practice optimal care, not standard of care."

— Brad Bale, M.D., internationally recognized expert in heart attack prevention

CARDIOVASCULAR DISEASE

The maximum amount of salt it's safe to eat
is 1,000 to 1,500 mg. a day.

If you stay in the produce aisle you don't have to worry—
otherwise read food labels!

Four grams of sugar is a teaspoon.

Read food labels-check the serving size
and then grams of sugar per serving.

Big Food has us hooked on salt, sugar, and fat.

Fruit juice is basically flavored sugar water.

We evolved to get our nutrients through chewing,
not through juicing, smoothies, pills, or supplements.

For a product to have fiber and whole grains, read the food label
(the ratio of total carbs to fiber should be 5:1 or less)
multiply the number for fiber by 5
the result should be greater than the number for total carbs.

TAKE CARE OF YOUR ENDOTHELIUM

The endothelium is an organ, one-cell thick, that lines our arteries. It is the largest organ in our body and if spread out it would cover the area of six tennis courts. In their book *Beat the Heart Attack Gene,* Bale and Doneen state that "some doctors call the endothelium the 'brain' of the arteries because it plays a vital role in regulating blood pressure and other vessel activities." Doctors used to think that damaged endothelium was an inevitable result of aging, but now we know that if people lead an optimal lifestyle, their endothelium remains "pristine" into their 90s and beyond, irrespective of their genetics. People who mistreat their endothelium end up with stiff, hardened arteries that have lost their elasticity. These people are prone to high blood pressure, heart attacks and strokes, peripheral vascular disease that affects their legs, kidney failure, erectile dysfunction, and dementia.

The endothelium makes nitric oxide, which causes arteries to dilate and keeps them healthy. Researchers can determine which factors damage endothelium and which ones support endothelial health by putting monitors on subjects' brachial arteries (upper arm), feeding them different foods and seeing if the arteries dilate (good) or constrict (bad). Coronary (heart) arteries can be studied during open heart surgery.

Here are some things that increase production of endothelial nitric oxide, resulting in arterial dilation:

- Moderate exercise
- Plant-based foods, particularly arugula, rhubarb, cilantro, butter leaf lettuce, mesclun greens, basil, beet greens, oak leaf lettuce, Swiss chard, and beets (per Dr. Greger in his book *How Not to Die*)
- Turmeric, walnuts, potassium, decaf coffee, green tea (if you put milk or creamer in your coffee or tea, the benefit is negated)
- Alcohol-free red wine
- Vinegar
- ACE (angiotensin converting enzyme) inhibitors such as lisinopril and ramipril, and to a lesser extent ARBs (angiotensin receptor blockers) such as losartan, both of which are used to treat high blood pressure

Here are a few of the things that have been shown to damage endothelium, causing arteries to stiffen and constrict:

- Sedentary lifestyle
- Prolonged sitting
- Too much exercise, such as running marathons and ultramarathons
- Smoking
- Animal products, including meat, fish, dairy, and eggs (Don't believe it? Go to Dr. Greger's well-referenced book *How Not to Die* or his website *nutrition-facts.org*)
- All added oils, including olive and coconut
- Salt (sodium)
- Caffeinated coffee (it's not the caffeine that makes this unhealthy per Dr. Greger, but some undetermined compound that is removed in the decaf process)
- Alcohol (sorry, I'm just the messenger)
- Sugar
- Inflammation, such as rheumatoid arthritis and dental/gum issues

As a particularly popular treat, chocolate deserves special mention. Unfortunately, chocolate is usually combined with milk and sugar, which harm the endothelium, and milk chocolate has lots of calories. But dark chocolate and pure, unprocessed chocolate in the form of cacao powder (which is minimally processed) and nibs improve endothelial function. Bale and Doneen recommend 1 or 2 squares (7–10 grams) of at least 72 percent dark chocolate a day. The healthiest way to get the benefits of chocolate is to eat a teaspoon of cacao powder a day, which I put in my tea in the morning. Eating a few cacao nibs a day is another healthy option. The powder and the nibs are more bitter than what you're used to when you eat or drink chocolate, but you quickly get used to the taste.

The bottom line is this: Being kind to your endothelium has many health benefits, including preventing the main cause of death and disability in countries on a Western diet: heart attacks and strokes respectively. You can find many tasty healthy recipes in cookbooks such as *Oh She Glows, Isa Does It,* and *Thug Kitchen,* (this one has some off-color language). Sure, you'll miss salt, sugar, and fat at first but after 10–14 days you will lose your taste for them.

CARDIOVASCULAR DISEASE

A MIRACLE?
NO, JUST A CHANGE IN DIET

Michael Greger, M.D., is the author of *nutritionfacts.org* and a book called *How Not to Die*. He is one of the few physicians who is truly an expert in nutrition, having made it his life's work to stay on the cutting edge of nutrition research and disseminate the information to lay people and health professionals. In the preface of his book, he tells the interesting story of what drove him to get into this.

At age 65, his beloved grandmother had developed end-stage atherosclerosis (hardening of the arteries). She had angina—blockages in her coronary arteries that caused her to have chest pain just walking across the room. She also had peripheral vascular disease, meaning arterial blockages in her legs, which caused leg pain after walking short distances. She had several bypass and stent procedures, but her vascular surgeons eventually couldn't do any more to help her and sent her home from the hospital in a wheel chair, to die.

About that time, *60 Minutes* did a health tip on the new Pritikin Diet, which was a plant-based, whole foods, low-fat diet which had been shown to reverse atherosclerosis. Dr. Greger's grandmother traveled to California, where the inpatient Pritikin Center was located. Three weeks after starting the program she went from not being able to walk across the room to being able to walk 10 miles. She stuck with the plant-based diet and lived to 96! There are lots of similar stories in the plant-based literature. We now know that atherosclerosis can resolve if we quit feeding it with the meat and dairy-based Western Diet, such as the S.A.D. (Standard American Diet). Obviously, the blockages in Dr. Greger's grandmother's arteries didn't resolve in 3 weeks, but as soon as she changed her diet, her endothelium—the organ that lines our arteries—started producing artery-dilating nitric oxide.

Understandably, this is what drove young Dr. Greger to go to medical school and help people prevent and treat disease through nutrition. Most medical schools have very little training in nutrition, if any, but he chose one that had at least some.

Why hasn't prevention and treatment of disease through lifestyle gained much traction in the U.S.? Unfortunately, instead of a health care system in this country we have developed an expensive disease management system—based on treating disease with pills and procedures rather than preventing and treating disease with lifestyle modification. There are many interests benefiting financially from the status quo—particularly hospitals, insurance companies, the pharmaceutical and medical device industries, and physician specialist societies (read *Mistreated, Why We Think We're Getting Good Health Care—And Why We're Usually Wrong*).

CARDIOVASCULAR DISEASE

"Leafy greens such as romaine lettuce, kale, collards, Swiss chard, and spinach are the most nutrient-dense of all foods."

– Joel Fuhrman, M.D.

HOW TO BOOST YOUR CHILD'S IMMUNE SYSTEM

The average young child gets 7 to 10 viral upper respiratory infections a year, often complicated by ear infections. To understand how you can boost your child's immunity, you need to have a basic understanding of the immune system. In his book *How Not to Die*, Dr. Greger notes that "the first layer of protection against intruders are physical surface barriers" like your skin, the mucus membranes that line your nose and mouth, and the layer of cells that line the intestines. The next layer of defense is white blood cells called neutrophils that attack viruses and bacteria; another type of white blood cells known as B cells make antibodies that "home in like smart bombs" when pathogens appear; and "natural killer cells that put your cells out of their misery if they become cancerous or infected with a virus."

What factors boost your child's immunity?
- Vaginal secretions a baby gets during a vaginal birth (They colonize their gut with "good" bacteria that help fight infection. If the child is delivered by caesarian, vaginal secretions wiped on the baby's mouth accomplish the same thing.)
- Breastfeeding until age 2
- Immunizations
- In older children, adequate sleep, stress reduction, and physical activity (but not too much such as intense training for competitive sports)
- Eating fruit and vegetables
- Avoidance of unnecessary antibiotics

Some examples of how eating fruit and vegetables improve immune function are the following: Kale dripped on white blood cells in a petri dish in the lab increases antibody production. Intensely-colored fruit such as berries boost numbers of killer cells. Cruciferous vegetables such as broccoli, cauliflower, brussels sprouts, and cabbage contain compounds that boost intestinal defenses. Mushrooms boost blood levels of IgA antibodies.

The gut microbiome consists of billions of bacteria and has implications for several aspects of our health, including immunity. So-called pre-biotics such as fiber feed health-promoting bacteria in our gut microbiome—pre-biotics are found in plants but not animal products. Antibiotics cause bacteria in our body to become antibiotic-resistant. Antibiotics also change our gut microbiome from health-promoting to disease-promoting. Both of these antibiotic side effects reduce immunity.

Joel Fuhrman, M.D., is one of the giants in plant-based nutrition. He wrote a book called *Disease-Proof Your Child.* In it he mentions that American children eat less than 2 percent of their diet from natural plant foods such as fruits and vegetables and that "toddlers between ages one and two eat no fruits and vegetables at all." Your mother had it right when she said "eat your veggies and go outside and play."

"Overall, our population is in the worst shape it's ever been.
Children are in terrible shape.
We have absolutely unprecedented numbers
of obese and overweight children—one in three now.
A generation ago it was something like one in ten."

- Neal Barnard, M.D.

HOW TO PREVENT YOUR CHILD FROM DEVELOPING THE CHRONIC DISEASES THAT AFFLICT SO MANY AMERICAN ADULTS

Many years ago a statistician figured out that a Happy Meal at McDonald's causes the same adverse health effects in a child as smoking 2 cigarettes. No parent would offer their child cigarettes, but many let their children eat unhealthy food.

Most American adults die from heart attacks and strokes, and the number 2 killer is cancer. Type 2 diabetes is becoming more prevalent as obesity increases in America, leading to complications such as vision loss, cardiovascular disease, kidney failure, and nerve problems.

The first signs of heart disease are streaks of fat in the endothelium—the delicate organ that lines the inside of our arteries. Fatty streaks have been observed in newborns of mothers with very high cholesterols, and in infants and toddlers who are on an animal-based diet. In the Korean and Vietnam wars, autopsies were done on young soldiers killed in battle—the American soldiers had hardening of the arteries but the Asian soldiers didn't. This was due to differences in diet, not genetics, because when Koreans and Vietnamese come to the U.S. and eat the S.A.D. (Standard American Diet), they get heart disease just like the rest of us. So as Dr. Esselstyn (*Forks Over Knives* documentary, author of the book *Prevent and Reverse Heart Disease*) says, heart disease is a food-borne illness, that doesn't occur in people who are plant-based all their lives.

Cancer is the second most common cause of death in adults on a Western diet, and it often starts years before people are diagnosed with it. We have billions of cells in our bodies, some of which are always mutating. Plants have micronutrients that improve our immunity and kill off these abnormal cells, preventing cancer down the road. According to Joel Fuhrman, M.D., in his book *Disease-Proof Your Child*, there is a strong link between lack of fruit and vegetables (along with eating meat and dairy products, refined food, and sugar) and "later-life cancers." There is also a link between industrial pollutants such as pesticides and later-life cancer. In this regard it is important to know that meat has 14 times and dairy 5.5 times the toxins than eating plants, at the bottom of the food chain.

Type 1 diabetes that usually starts in childhood is an autoimmune disease, which is less common in people who are plant-based. The more common type 2 diabetes is related to obesity, and is now seen in overweight children (it used to be called "adult onset diabetes"). Kids who eat lots of fruit and veggies are much less apt to be overweight and to have type 2 diabetes.

According to Dr. Fuhrman, "American children … eat less than 2 percent of their diet from natural plant foods such as fruits and vegetables." This does not bode well for their future health.

"Eating a high-nutrient diet
actually makes you more satisfied with less food,
and actually gives the ability
to enjoy food more without overeating."

– Joel Fuhrman, M.D.

HOW TO GET KIDS TO EAT THEIR VEGGIES

Those of us who have children and grandchildren know that the big question is: How do we get kids to eat fruit and veggies?

Michael Greger, M.D. has the following evidence-based suggestions:

- Children eat more fruits and veggies if their parents do—so parents, eat both.
- "Simply having healthy foods out and available can boost intake," even when unhealthy food is also available such as at a birthday party.
- Cut veggies into slices, sticks, or stars.
- Put Elmo stickers on veggies. In one study this "swayed 50 percent of children to choose broccoli over a chocolate bar."
- Call foods by kid-friendly names such as "X-ray vision carrots" or "power punch broccoli."
- Dip veggies in unprocessed peanut butter.
- Veggies such as broccoli, cauliflower, tomatoes, squash, and zucchini can be added covertly to various entrees.

In his book *Disease-Proof Your Child*, Joel Fuhrman, M.D. has a chapter called "Reforming the Picky Eater," which includes the following suggestions:

- Permit only healthy food in the house.
- Persist in getting kids to try new foods, which studies show often takes 8 to 15 attempts.
- Offer only healthy snacks such as fruit, vegetables, bean and nut dips, wholesome soups, and raw, unsalted nuts.
- Avoid unwholesome treats, e.g. "if you eat all your veggies you can have ice cream for dessert."

Here are a couple of my own suggestions, from years of being a parent and grandparent:

- Organic edamame (soy beans) are a healthy snack kids will eat. You can buy bags of frozen edamame at most grocery stores.

- Berries are another healthy snack that kids will eat.
- Carrot sticks, sweet peppers, and celery sticks dipped in hummus with no added oil (e.g. the Engine 2 Plant Strong brand at Whole Foods, or make your own), makes a healthy snack.
- If your child participates in sports, tell them about all the elite athletes who are eating fruit, veggies, and whole grains to enhance performance (you get the most nutrients per calorie that way).
- If you're a grandparent, it's fine to spoil your grandkids a little, but their current and future health suffers if you use unhealthy food to spoil them.

CHILDREN

"Fast food leads to a slow death."

- Greg Feinsinger, M.D.

(Referring to the chronic diseases brought on by fast food.)

IS A VEGAN DIET SAFE FOR YOUNG CHILDREN?

The short answer is yes, with a few caveats. The science tells us that the healthiest diet is one rich in fruit, vegetables, and whole grains, with no salt, sugar, or added oil. This is the diet that humans ate as our genome developed over 20 million years, and our jaw and GI structures are those of plant-eaters. But parents often ask if this diet is safe for young children, because the meat, dairy, egg, and fish industries have committed false advertising for decades, convincing us that children need their products to grow up to be big, strong, and smart.

One thing we know for sure is that the S.A.D. (Standard American Diet) is not good for the developing human fetus if the mother is eating it, for children of any age, and for adults. The S.A.D. is high in trans and saturated fat, processed carbohydrates, sugar and salt, and oil, all of which are addictive. Most meat contains antibiotics. And since meat, dairy, eggs, and fish are at the top of the food chain they are loaded with industrial pollutants and other toxins compared to plants. Not only are these products unnecessary for optimal childhood health, but they also contribute to many childhood diseases such as asthma, and to most of the chronic diseases that eventually afflict many American adults: obesity; diabetes; hypertension; high cholesterol; cardiovascular disease; autoimmune diseases such as type 1 diabetes, ulcerative colitis and lupus; inflammatory diseases such as asthma and rheumatoid arthritis; osteoporosis; dementia; and many types of cancer including breast, prostate, and colon.

To answer the question posed in the title, let's start with fetal health: We've all heard that pregnant women should avoid alcohol and cigarettes and certain fish. But optimal fetal health is achieved by avoiding all animal (including fish) and dairy products, and by the mother eating a balanced plant-based diet with adequate omega-3. The healthiest food for an infant is breast milk, and authorities such as Dr. Fuhrman recommend breastfeeding until age 2, with slow introduction of plant-based solids starting at 6 months. The content of breast milk is influenced by what the mother eats, so for optimal infant health the mother should eat a plant-based diet.

Both animal and plant products have all the macronutrients babies, toddlers, and older children need: protein, carbohydrates, and fat. It's a misconception that a plant-based diet is restrictive—what is restrictive is an animal-based diet, which lacks the fiber, the vitamins and minerals, and the thousands of health-promoting micronutrients that plants contain (vitamins in pill form or added to food products cannot do what natural vitamins in food we eat can do, and can even cause harm).

There are a few caveats:

- It's important that plant-based children eat some nuts and seeds including hemp or ground flaxseeds every day, so that their bodies can convert these things to omega-3 (healthy fat). Another good source of healthy fat is avocados.
- To be on the safe side, a daily omega-3 supplement is wise.
- Vitamin B12 is made from bacteria in dirt, and due to treated water and pre-washed produce, we don't eat much dirt these days. A vegan diet can lead to B12 deficiency, so anyone on a plant-based diet should take a B12 supplement daily.
- This has nothing to do with being plant-based, but most humans are deficient in vitamin D, and starting in infancy should take a D3 supplement (as the human genome was developing, people were running around equatorial Africa mainly naked, and they had much higher vitamin D levels compared to people today).

For more information, including the doses of omega-3, B12, and D3 for various ages, read *Disease-Proof Your Child,* by Joel Fuhrman, M.D. Another good source is *How Not to Die*, by Michael Greger, M.D., and his website *nutritionfacts.org.* You can talk to your doctor, but keep in mind that very few doctors, including pediatricians, know much if anything about nutrition; one study showed that people off the street knew more about nutrition than doctors. I didn't either until I read *The China Study* and watched *Forks Over Knives.* Talking to dietitians can be problematic because their national organization is heavily funded by Big Food.

CHILDREN

CHOLESTEROL, THE GOOD AND THE BAD

Cholesterol is the precursor of bile acids and steroid hormones and is a constituent of cell membranes. We need cholesterol, but high levels cause problems. Most of our cholesterol is produced by our liver, but some comes from food we eat. A typical cholesterol test, called a "lipid panel," includes a total cholesterol; LDL (L for lousy) cholesterol; HDL (H for healthy) cholesterol; and triglycerides. I tell patients to think of their LDL as garbage in their arteries and HDL as garbage trucks—they will have problems with their arteries if they have too much garbage or too few garbage trucks. Some doctors tell their patients that they don't have to fast to have a lipid panel drawn, but triglycerides tend to be high in the non-fasting state, so I tell my patients to fast for six hours (water is okay).

There are cholesterol skeptics out there who claim on the Internet and elsewhere that high cholesterol is not related to disease, but this belief is not based on sound science. High cholesterol and especially high LDL are clearly associated with atherosclerosis ("hardening of the arteries"), which is the cause of heart attacks, strokes, peripheral vascular disease (blockages in leg arteries), chronic kidney disease, erectile dysfunction, and dementia. Cholesterol is present in arterial plaque, and electron microscope photos show cholesterol crystals poking through the capsule that surrounds plaque, causing plaque rupture, resulting in heart attacks and strokes. There is a genetic abnormality called familial hyperlipidemia, where sufferers have extremely high cholesterol levels, and some children with this disease die in their teens from heart attacks.

On the other hand, half of people with heart attacks have normal cholesterol. The U.S. guidelines recommend that normal total cholesterol levels should be less than 200; LDL less than 100; triglycerides less than 150; HDL greater than 40 in a male or post-menopausal female; and HDL greater than 50 in a pre-menopausal female. The guidelines also recommend that if a person has had a heart attack their LDL should be less than 70. Heart attack prevention doctors (who with some exceptions aren't cardiologists) disagree with the latter guideline, because around 20 percent of people die from their first heart attack. Therefore, we advise patients to have a carotid IMT or coronary calcium score to see if they have plaque in their arteries. If they do, they are at risk for a heart attack or stroke and we recommend an LDL of less than 70.

Populations who are on a lifelong plant-based, whole food diet with no salt, sugar, or added oil don't get atherosclerosis and therefore are heart attack-proof. Their total cholesterols are less than 150, LDLs are in the 30s and 40s, and triglycerides less than 70. These are the levels in human newborns and in other mammals that don't get atherosclerosis. So, these are the levels plant-based doctors want in our patients.

The usual lipid panel measures the level of LDL, but a more meaningful measurement is the LDL particle number (the number of LDL particles per unit of blood). Small, dense LDL particles are more dangerous than large ones (b-bs compared to ping-pong balls). Another blood test that heart attack prevention doctors always order is Lp(a), which is a particularly harmful type of LDL that responds to niacin and to a plant-based diet, but not to statins. Finally, heart disease is not all about cholesterol—inflammation plays a role, particularly inflammation due to tooth or gum disease. Heart attack prevention doctors often order an "advanced lipid profile" through the Berkeley or Cleveland Heart Lab, which includes all the above tests plus inflammatory markers that measure inflammation of the endothelial lining of the arteries and of plaque: MPO and LpPLA2 respectively. The commonly-ordered hsCRP—highly sensitive C-reactive protein—is a non-specific test for inflammation anywhere in the body.

Your liver makes more LDL if you eat saturated fat found in oils and in animal products. A plant-based diet improves lipid levels, often dramatically, and most studies show this diet is 98 percent effective in preventing heart attacks. Statins prevent the liver from making so much LDL cholesterol, but are only 30 percent effective in preventing heart attacks. If triglycerides are even mildly elevated and HDL on the low side, diabetes or pre-diabetes are almost always the cause.

In their book *Beat the Heart Attack Gene,* Bale and Doneen recommend that anyone with plaque in their arteries take a statin drug, no matter what their total cholesterol or LDL are. If you don't want to do that or have had side effects from statins, try Amla (Indian gooseberry), which has been shown to be very effective in lowering cholesterol, inflammation, and blood sugar. (Search Amla on Dr. Greger's website *nutritionfacts.org*.) Order Amla on the Internet, but be sure it's organic and from a reputable company.

CHOLESTEROL

COMMON COLD

Viruses that cause the common cold (a.k.a. upper respiratory infection, or U.R.I.) become more prevalent as the weather gets colder. Typical symptoms include nasal stuffiness or runny nose, mild ear and facial discomfort, low grade fever, mild aching, mild sore throat, mild generalized aching, and mild cough. Sometimes the nasal drainage becomes a little yellowish or greenish, which is from the white blood cells that fight off the virus; this does not indicate a bacterial infection. Antibiotics can be life-saving for serious bacterial infections such as pneumonia and meningitis, but are not effective against viruses, so don't request them for cold symptoms.

Typically, colds resolve in 7–10 days. Across-the-counter cold remedies are often associated with side effects (decongestants make many people feel wired, antihistamines cause drowsiness), and many people would rather have the cold symptoms than these side effects. The safest medication to take for mild fever and aching is acetaminophen.

Rarely, bacterial complications result from a cold. The following symptoms need to be checked out immediately: High fever and/or shaking chills could mean a blood infection. Chest pain, shortness of breath, or difficulty breathing could mean pneumonia. A severe headache and/or stiff neck could mean meningitis.

A sinus infection, while not usually serious, usually occurs several days after onset of the U.R.I. symptoms. It is manifested by pain in the cheek and teeth, usually on one side, and thick dark yellow or green nasal drainage all day long (not just first thing in the morning). A bacterial ear infection is usually manifested by worsening and persistent pain in one ear.

Nothing has really been shown to prevent colds, other than keeping your immune system in top shape by healthy diet, adequate sleep, and stress reduction.

SORE THROAT

Mild sore throats are usually due to viral infections such as the common cold, in which case they are accompanied by other cold symptoms. If you have a moderate to severe sore throat, without a runny nose or cough or other cold symptoms, you need to see if it is due to the strep bacteria, because if left untreated strep throat can result in rheumatic fever or a kidney disease called glomerulonephritis. Typically, strep throat is also associated with sore, tender neck glands and a white exudate in the throat.

Most labs allow people to obtain a rapid strep test without an order from a physician, with results available in minutes. Usually, if the rapid test is negative an overnight throat culture is done, and occasionally this will be positive even if the rapid test is negative. In any case, if your test is positive for strep, see or contact your provider, because you need an antibiotic. Penicillin is usually used, or erythromycin in the case of penicillin allergy.

"The whiter your bread,
the sooner you're dead."

– Joel Fuhrman, M.D.

(Referring to the dangers of refined food.)

WHAT IS THE SAFEST COOKWARE?

The University of California, *Berkeley Wellness Letter* has a useful article about the pros and cons of various types of cookware. Here are some of the highlights:

TEFLON
- Teflon, which prevents sticking, was discovered by a DuPont chemist in 1938. It is a brand name for polytetrafluoroethylene (PTFE), and other companies have developed other brands.
- Fumes from heating PTFE-coated pots and pans to temperatures over 660 degrees can cause symptoms in humans and death in pet birds.
- There is no evidence that ingesting PTFE flakes from old cookware causes cancer. However, there are concerns about cancer and hormone disruption from another chemical, called PFOA, which until 2015 was used in the manufacturing of PTFE and which persists in our environment and our bodies.
- The replacements for PFOA may not be any safer (we don't know yet). The nonprofit advocacy group The Environmental Working Group advises consumers to avoid all nonstick cookware and kitchen utensils.
- At the very least, avoid high temperatures with stick-free cookware, and replace it when it starts to deteriorate.

ALUMINUM
- Aluminum cookware can scratch and stain easily and can give acidic food such as tomato sauce a bitter taste because aluminum leaches into the food.
- In his book *Power Foods For The Brain,* Dr. Neal Barnard points out that there is still concern that aluminum ingestion may be linked to Alzheimer's.
- Ideally you should avoid aluminum cookware because you don't want to risk brain health.
- If you do buy it, buy the anodized variety, which has a harder surface. However, if labeled nonstick, it may contain PFTE-related compounds.
- At the very least, avoid acid foods such as tomatoes with aluminum cookware.

CAST IRON
- To maintain a cast-iron pan you have to rub oil on the surface, and a well-seasoned pan is fairly stick-free.
- Iron leaches into acidic food.
- Although we need some iron in our diet, we get plenty from what we eat (including if you are plant-based). Too much iron causes free radicals to form, which contribute to aging, cancer, heart disease, and other health problems. According to Dr. Barnard, there is a link between high blood iron levels and Alzheimer's.
- Cast-iron cookware should be dried as soon as it is washed and should not be put in the dishwasher to avoid rusting (i.e. oxidation).

CERAMIC-COATED
- It is non-stick but contains no PTFE or PFOA, is heat-stable and flake-resistant.
- It is therefore thought to be free of health and environmental concerns.
- However, some products may use nanoparticle coatings, and the long-term health and environmental effects of nanoparticles are unknown.

COPPER
- Copper can leach into food unless it's lined with stainless steel.
- We need a small amount of copper in our diet but too much causes health problems. Dr. Barnard talks in his book about evidence linking copper to Alzheimer's, so it's best to avoid copper cookware.

STAINLESS STEEL
- Stainless steel cookware does not react with food and doesn't rust.
- Some have an inner core of copper or aluminum that helps food cook more uniformly, but this should not be a problem as long as the surface is stainless steel.

GLASS
- Pyrex is the best-known brand and was introduced over a century ago.
- Glass is inert, does not react with food, and poses no known health or environmental problems.

So, the bottom line is this: Avoid copper, aluminum, and iron cookware for optimal health. Ideally use glass and stainless steel for cooking. Ceramic cookware is safe if it is not coated with nanoparticles. If sticking is a problem with these safe options, a small amount of oil rubbed on the surface solves the problem, though keep in mind, added oils cause several health problems and carcinogens form when oils reach their smoke point. So, it's better to use vegetable broth, water, wine, or soy sauce to prevent sticking.

COOKWARE

THE MOUTH-HEART CONNECTION

It's becoming increasingly apparent that there is a strong connection between your mouth and your arteries. One obvious connection is the relationship between the food you put in your mouth and the health of your heart. One of my favorite quotes, by Ann Wigmore, is this: "The food you eat can be the safest, most powerful medicine or the slowest form of poison." So if you eat the S.A.D. (Standard American Diet), you are slowly poisoning yourself.

In their book *Beat The Heart Attack Gene,* Brad Bale, M.D. and Amy Doneen, N.P. PhD note that there is recent evidence that diseases of the teeth (cavities, root canal infections) and gums (periodontal disease) can cause formation of plaque in the arteries, and can also cause the inflammation of arterial plaque that leads to rupture—the cause of heart attacks and most strokes. Dental issues explain why some people have heart attacks and strokes without having the usual risk factors such as high cholesterol, hypertension, positive family history, and diabetes.

Heart attacks and strokes are not all about cholesterol, and the missing piece of the puzzle is inflammation. People with inflammatory diseases such as rheumatoid arthritis are at 7 times the risk for a cardiovascular event. For the rest of us, inflammation is often dental. When Bale and Doneen see a patient for heart attack prevention, they routinely order a Cleveland Heart Lab test, which includes inflammatory markers. Highly sensitive C-reactive protein is a non-specific inflammatory marker (an elevation could mean vascular inflammation but could also mean arthritis or other inflammation). The myeloperoxidase (MPO) test is for inflammation of the endothelial lining of the arteries; the LpPLA2 (PLAC2) test is for inflammation of arterial plaque, which can lead to plaque rupture/heart attack or stroke. If the MPO or PLAC2 are elevated, Bale and Doneen refer the patient to a dentist who is well-versed in the mouth-heart connection.

If you want to prevent a heart attack or stroke, good dental hygiene is very important: brush after meals, floss correctly (don't just snap the floss between your teeth but rather the floss should form a C-shape on each side of each tooth) at least after your evening meal, and use a water pick after your evening meal and ideally after every meal.

Bleeding from your gums is a sign of gum disease, and if this occurs see your dentist right away. See your dentist if you have any pain in your teeth, although you can have significant tooth infections without any symptoms so you should see your dentist routinely and have X-rays done periodically. Bale and Doneen say that anyone who has a heart attack or stroke should have a complete dental checkup, including a saliva test called MyPeriPath, which shows the balance between the different bacteria in the mouth, and if "bad bacteria" have taken over.

I have taken the Bale-Doneen Method (of heart attack prevention) preceptorship, and recently attended their 2-day preceptorship reunion. Interestingly, over half the attendees were dentists, who seem to be understanding the mouth-heart connection before physicians are.

"Blueberries, strawberries and blackberries
are true super foods."

– Joel Fuhrman, M.D.

DENTAL

DEPRESSION IS COMMON, TREATABLE

Everyone feels sad at times, especially following a loss. Depression is different: it lasts longer and is more disabling. It can occur in children, the elderly, and everyone in between. Depression is common, affecting 7 percent of Americans (15 million) at any given time. It is the most common cause of disability between the ages of 15 and 45.

The common symptoms of depression are: prolonged sadness, loss of energy, irritability, social withdrawal, loss of interest in activities that previously were pleasurable, early-morning awakening or other sleep disturbances including sleeping too much, loss of appetite, heightened sensitivity to pain, numb emotions, difficulty concentrating and making decisions, unwarranted feelings of guilt, and thoughts of dying. The one symptom that everyone with depression has is absence of "zest for life." In children, depression can manifest as behavioral problems at home and a drop in school performance. In the elderly, depression can mimic dementia. This health tip is about unipolar depression, as opposed to bipolar depression, which is characterized by depressive lows alternating with abnormal highs.

A person with a family history of depression, anxiety, or substance abuse is at higher risk for depression, so there can be a genetic component. Although the biology of depression is not completely understood, low levels of brain neurotransmitters such as serotonin, norepinephrine, and dopamine seem to play a role. Anti-depressants boost levels of these neurotransmitters.

Depression can adversely affect other people, including co-workers, friends, and family members. Clear thinking is impaired in depressed people, who often think they'd feel better if they just had a different job or a different spouse or if they moved to another location; for this reason, depressed people should avoid making important, life-changing decisions. Depression can be deadly, and suicide affects those left behind for the rest of their lives. In 2014, 42,826 Americans lost their lives due to suicide, and firearms were used in half of these cases. Suicide is a permanent fix for a treatable, temporary problem, and what's often forgotten in the gun debate is that if there is a gun handy, depressed people are more apt to make an impulsive decision to kill themselves than if they had to figure out another way.

Depression is treatable, through counseling and/or anti-depressants. Unfortunately,

80 percent of depressed people don't seek help, especially macho men. Many people tolerate anti-depressants well, although some complain of side effects. However, the side effects are usually mild and beat having depression. Sleep apnea can cause depression and is common; treating it can improve and resolve depression. (The screening test for this is inexpensive and easy: wear an oximeter on your finger all night, which records your oxygen level and pulse rate.)

There is clear evidence that regular exercise—both aerobic and strength training—helps prevent and treat depression. An anti-inflammatory diet high in antioxidants also helps. This means plant-based, whole (unprocessed) food with no added oil, salt, or sugar, as opposed to an animal-based diet, which causes inflammation. Specific foods that have been proven to help prevent and treat depression are nuts, seeds, legumes, greens, coffee, tomatoes, carrots, and several spices including saffron. A local psychiatrist once told me that his patients respond better to anti-depressants if they are on a plant-based diet. Depressed people should avoid alcohol, which worsens sleep problems and depression. For more details about nutrition and depression, search "depression" on Dr. Greger's website *nutritionfacts.org* or read the chapter on depression in his book *How Not to Die*.

During my 42 years of family practice, I saw countless people with depression. When I saw them back for follow-up a week after starting them on an anti-depressant, most felt much better. In summary, If you have symptoms of depression for more than a week or two, you don't have to continue to suffer. Try the above lifestyle changes first, but if you aren't feeling better within several days, see your primary care provider or a mental health expert. Psychologists and counselors can't prescribe medication but PCPs and psychiatrists can. Counseling plus anti-depressants have been shown to be the most effective, if lifestyle changes aren't enough.

"The food you eat can be either the safest
and most powerful form of medicine,
or the slowest form of poison."

– Ann Wigmore

(If you are eating the S.A.D.—Standard American Diet—
you are slowly poisoning yourself.)

DEPRESSION

WHAT WE EAT CAN AFFECT OUR MOOD

Dr. Michael Greger's book *How Not to Die* and his website *nutritionfacts.org*, cite studies that show that people who live a plant-based, whole (unprocessed) food lifestyle have less tension, anxiety, depression, anger, hostility, and fatigue. Here are some examples:

- Removing meat, fish, poultry, and eggs from the diet of depressed people improves mood scores in just 2 weeks.
- Diets high in unprocessed carbs and low in fat and protein decrease anxiety and depression.
- A study of a U.S. corporation showed that employees at 10 different sites noted less depression and anxiety and had increased productivity after going plant-based.
- Eating vegetables just 3 times a week improved depression scores by 60 percent in another study.
- Consumption of beverages with sugar increased the risk of depression, as did artificial sweeteners.

Here are some of the reasons that eating plants help prevent and treat depression:

- Arachidonic acid: Our bodies make this omega-6 fatty acid, which causes the inflammation we need to promote healing after an injury. However, high levels caused by dietary intake inflame the nervous system, including the brain, which leads to depression. The 2 foods that are primarily responsible for high levels of arachidonic acid are poultry and eggs, although meat and fish also contribute. Arachidonic acid is not found in plants.
- Oxidative stress, which causes free radicals, plays a role in depression. Fruits and vegetables are loaded with antioxidants, particularly ones with intense flavor (herbs and spices, especially turmeric and amla) and color (e.g. greens, peppers, yams, berries). Animal products contain few to no antioxidants.
- Lycopenes are antioxidants found in tomatoes, watermelon, pink grapefruit, guava, and papaya, and high blood levels are associated with less depression.

- Low blood levels of folate are associated with depression. Greens and beans are good dietary sources of folate. Note that folic acid supplements don't help (natural folate isn't exactly the same thing as folic acid in supplements, plus we evolved to get our nutrients from the food we eat, not pills).
- Monoamines include the neurotransmitters serotonin and dopamine, which help prevent depression. Monoamine oxidase (MAO) is an enzyme that breaks down excess monoamines. Depressed people have a defect in this regulatory mechanism, causing high levels of MAO, which results in low levels of the depression-preventing monoamines. Pharmaceutical companies have developed MAO inhibitors, but they can cause serious side effects. Several foods have natural, side-effect-free plant nutrients that inhibit MAO: apples, berries, grapes, kale, onions, green tea, cloves, oregano, cinnamon, and nutmeg.
- Tryptophan is a building block of serotonin, the "happiness hormone." According to Dr. Greger, foods with a high tryptophan-to-protein ratio help facilitate tryptophan transport into the brain: sesame, sunflower, pumpkin, and butternut squash seeds.

In conclusion, the same plant-based foods that are necessary for optimal physical health also cause optimal mental health. This is not surprising, because the human genome evolved over some 20 million years when pre-humans were herbivores. Also, our jaw and GI structures are those of herbivores rather than carnivores. This is not to say that all plant-based people are free of depression. But plant-based nutrition can help prevent and treat depression. And being on a plant-based diet enhances the effect of anti-depressants.

"This spread of obesity
foreshadows an explosion in degenerative diseases,
such as diabetes, heart disease, and cancer
waiting to erupt in our children's future."

– Joel Fuhrman, M.D.

DEPRESSION

THE IMPORTANCE OF EARLY DIAGNOSIS AND REVERSAL OF PRE-DIABETES

There are 2 types of diabetes: type 1 and type 2. Type 1 is an autoimmune disorder that usually occurs in childhood or teenage years—often in thin people. Type 2 diabetes, or what we used to call adult onset diabetes, is what this tip will discuss. It is much more common than type 1, and more than 102 million Americans suffer from diabetes or pre-diabetes, although 34 million of them don't know it, either because they haven't had their blood sugar checked or because they were checked with unreliable tests. Type 2 diabetes usually occurs in people who are overweight, and now that many youngsters are over-weight and are developing diabetes, we can no longer call it "adult onset diabetes."

Diabetes is much more than a simple blood sugar problem because after several years, pre-diabetics and diabetics develop conditions such as eye damage; kidney fail-ure; nerve damage causing pain and numbness in the legs and feet; heart attacks and strokes; and peripheral vascular disease that can result in amputations. So, not only can diabetes shorten lifespan, but it also interferes with quality of life. Nobody wants to get diabetes, but what a lot of people don't realize is that a large percentage of type 2 di-abetes is preventable, and if it's already present it is reversible if caught early enough.

Years before diabetes is diagnosed—usually on the basis of an elevated fasting blood sugar—pre-diabetes is present, but unfortunately is under-diagnosed by providers at the stage where it could be reversed. What occurs first in most cases is central obesity, meaning heaviness around the middle. If you are a Caucasian, Hispanic, or African-American male and have a waist circumference of 40 inches or greater, or fe-male with a circumference of 35 inches or greater—measured at the area of greatest circumference rather than belt size—you almost certainly have pre-diabetes or diabetes. Asians and East Indians have lower cutoff points.

The problem with central obesity is that people with it have "visceral fat," meaning fat in and around their internal organs, as well as in their muscles. Visceral fat causes in-sulin resistance, where organs and tissues can't use insulin like they should. The pan-creas—which makes insulin—overcompensates for insulin resistance by pumping out more and more insulin, and eventually it wears out and diabetes is diagnosed. One of the first signs of insulin resistance is high triglycerides and low HDL (good cholesterol).

DIABETIES, PRE-DIABETES

If the triglyceride/HDL ratio is 3.5 or greater in Caucasians or 3.0 in Hispanics, insulin resistance is present.

Often diabetes isn't diagnosed until the fasting blood sugar becomes elevated, but it can take years before the fasting blood sugar becomes elevated, and by then, a lot of damage has occurred and may be difficult to reverse. Insulin resistance is the driver of 70 percent of cardiovascular disease, so if heart attack prevention doctors suspect it we recommend a 2-hour glucose tolerance test. The patient fasts for 12 hours, then drinks 75 grams of sugar in the lab, and has a blood sugar test 1 and 2 hours later. If the 1 hour is 125 or greater, or the 2 hour 120 or greater, the diagnosis of insulin resistance is confirmed. A1C is a blood test used to see what average blood sugars have been over the previous 3 months, and is a good blood test for monitoring control of diabetes once it's diagnosed. But according to Bale and Doneen, authors of *Beat the Heart Attack Gene*, A1C, is not a reliable test for diagnosing diabetes or pre-diabetes. If you think you might have diabetes or pre-diabetes, or have a positive family history, insist on the 2-hour glucose tolerance test.

People who exercise regularly and eat a plant-based, whole (unprocessed) food diet with no salt, sugar or added oil do not develop central obesity, insulin resistance/pre-diabetes, or type 2 diabetes. (People on this diet also have a much lower incidence of type 1 diabetes and other autoimmune diseases.)

There are medications that can treat and help prevent type 2 diabetes, but lifestyle modification is much more effective, costs nothing, and is free of side effects. There are no medications that prevent pre-diabetes.

"People love to spend money on books that tell them it's okay to continue eating the same unhealthy food."

– Caldwell Esselstyn, M.D.

DIABETIES, PRE-DIABETES

HEALTH CONCERNS ABOUT EATING MEAT

For decades, scientists have been aware of data linking meat intake (beef, lamb/mutton, pork, poultry) to a higher incidence of obesity, diabetes, hypertension, high cholesterol, cardiovascular disease (heart attacks and strokes), inflammatory diseases such as rheumatoid arthritis, autoimmune diseases such as M.S., dementia including Alzheimer's, and several forms of cancer. Recently, various medical organizations have been telling us to limit our intake of meat and ideally to avoid it altogether. The World Health Organization has declared red and processed meat (ham, bacon, hot dogs, sausage, lunch meat) to be class one carcinogens. An editorial in the March 2016 edition of the *American Family Physician* journal had the following title: "Eating Less Meat: A Healthy and Environmentally Responsible Dietary Choice."

The information for this health tip was obtained from several sources, including *How Not to Die* and *nutritionfacts.org* by Michael Greger, M.D.; *The End of Heart Disease* by Joel Fuhrman, M.D.; "Nutrition Action," published by the Center For Science in the Public Interest; and various communications from Neal Barnard, M.D., founding president of PCRM (Physician Committee for Responsible Medicine). Following are some of the health concerns associated with eating meat:

- In 2012 the results from two large Harvard studies indicated that consumption of red meat was associated with an increased risk of dying from heart disease and cancer, and an increased risk of early death.
- Meat contains saturated and trans fats, which cause your liver to make more LDL (bad cholesterol), which in turn contributes to atherosclerosis (hardening of the arteries), the cause of heart attacks and strokes.
- A meat-based diet is acidic and causes generalized inflammation, and this contributes to several diseases. In particular, meat inflames the endothelium, the delicate organ that lines our arteries, and this inflammation contributes to cardiovascular disease (heart attacks and strokes).
- One-third of Americans over age 64 have chronic kidney disease, and protein and fat from meat contribute to this condition.
- Eating poultry increases the risk of blood cancers such as leukemia, lymphoma, and myeloma, probably due to avian tumor-causing viruses.

- Often salt and water are injected into poultry and other meat carcasses to increase weight (meat is usually sold on a weight basis), and the salt contributes to hypertension. This injected meat can still be labeled as "100 percent natural."
- Unhealthy artificial dyes are often added to meat to improve appearance.
- Heterocyclic amines (HCAs) are a carcinogen formed when beef, pork, lamb, and poultry are cooked at high temperatures (pan frying, grilling, baking), resulting in an increased risk of cancer of the breast, colon, esophagus, lung, pancreas, prostate, and stomach.
- Farm animals and poultry are often injected with antibiotics, which contributes to antibiotic resistance; and with hormones that disrupt our natural human hormones.
- Heme iron in the blood and muscle of animals causes free radicals, which increase the risk of cardiovascular disease, cancer, and diabetes. Iron from vegetables (whole grains, legumes, nuts, seeds, dried fruit, green leafy vegetables) don't do this because absorption of non-heme (plant) iron is controlled by a feedback mechanism that limits absorption if iron levels are adequate.
- Salmonella and other harmful bacteria are present in uncooked meat, and can get on your kitchen counter and cooking utensils. Parasites can be present in meat, such as toxoplasmosis in pork. In 2014, Consumer Reports claimed that 97 percent of chicken breasts in grocery stores, 88 percent of ground beef, and 80 percent of pork chops are contaminated with animal fecal matter.
- Compared to plants, meat contains 14 times the amount of pesticides and other environmental toxins, because meat is at the top of the food chain. People with the highest levels of pollutants in their blood have 38 times the risk of diabetes.
- Fiber is important for optimal health, and meat contains no fiber.
- Animal protein triggers production of IGF1 (insulin growth factor), which in adults causes cancer cells to form and to spread.
- Animal proteins in meat contribute to formation of kidney stones.
- Red meat eaters have bacteria in their gut microbiomes that convert carnitine in meat to TMAO, which causes heart disease.
- Clearly the environmental impact associated with raising a pound of beef is huge compared to a pound of, say, kale.
- Watch the documentary *Food Inc.* to see the ethical problems with treatment of animals in factory farming.

Still not convinced? If you're going to continue to eat meat, wild game is the best because although it has cholesterol, it has much less cholesterol-raising saturated fat. Buying locally-grown meat addresses some of the environmental and the ethical treatment of animals concerns but still leaves the health concerns.

Why isn't this information more widely disseminated? Big Food is a huge lobby; tries to cast doubt on established science; has an undue influence on governmental committees and legislatures; influences the mass media; and influences the training of physicians, nurses, and dietitians. Dr. Greger points out that the American Dietetic Association receives millions of dollars annually from the beef, dairy, and egg industries.

"Why don't we just get our population healthier
so we don't need medical care?"

– Joel Fuhrman, M.D.

DIET—WHAT WE SHOULD AVOID FOR OPTIMAL HEALTH

FOR OPTIMAL HEALTH, AVOID SEAFOOD

Health concerns about seafood have been covered in other health tips, so this will be short. Following are the major concerns:

- Seafood is an animal protein, and in *The China Study*—the largest study on nutrition ever done—the people in China who were too poor to afford to eat animal protein didn't have all the chronic diseases we suffer from in societies on a Western diet (obesity, hypertension, diabetes, cardiovascular disease, cancer, etc.).
- Seafood is at the top of the food chain compared to eating plants, and therefore essentially all of it is contaminated by environmental toxins such as heavy metals and PCBs.
- People who eat seafood are more apt to be obese.
- Grilling seafood can result in the same carcinogens that are associated with grilling meat.
- Uncooked seafood can be a source of parasites, such as fish tapeworm in uncooked fish.
- Due to most of our oceans being overfished and to climate change, fish are becoming less abundant.

GOT MILK?
HEALTH CONCERNS ABOUT EATING DAIRY

Cows' milk is meant for baby cows, which are weaned after several months, so even cows don't drink milk after a certain age. Following are some of the reasons you should avoid dairy products. This is settled science, even though Big Dairy does its best to sow seeds of doubt.

- All dairy products have saturated fat, which raises LDL (bad cholesterol) and inflames the endothelium that lines our arteries, resulting in increased risk of heart attacks and strokes.
- Saturated fat also increases risk of obesity, insulin resistance/pre-diabetes, type 2 diabetes, and early death.
- Milk and cheese increase the risk of prostate cancer, probably due to IGF1 (insulin growth factor). IGF1 is important in the growth of baby mammals, but high levels in human adults stimulate cancer onset and spread.
- In his book *How Not to Die*, Dr. Michael Greger points out that all animal products contain sex steroid hormones such as estrogen, particularly now that cows are often milked throughout their pregnancies, "leading to hormone-related conditions such as acne, diminished male reproductive potential, and premature puberty."
- Your intake of toxins is increased markedly if you eat at the top of the food chain, i.e. animal products versus plants. Dr. Greger says that it is estimated that for every glass of milk you drink a day the risk of Parkinson's disease increases by 17 percent, due to neurotoxins.
- It may seem counterintuitive given the "Got Milk" advertising campaign, but dairy intake is associated with an increased risk of osteoporosis and fractures. The best way to get calcium is by eating plants such as leafy greens, beans including tofu, bok choy, broccoli, collard greens, kale, and sweet potatoes.
- Dr. Frank Sacks showed in the 1970s that milk intake raises blood pressure, irrespective of weight gain.
- Dairy and other animal products cause acidic urine, resulting in more kidney stones.

DIET—WHAT WE SHOULD AVOID FOR OPTIMAL HEALTH

- The food industry prioritizes big profits over your health, and has people hooked on salt, sugar, and fat. Often sugar and salt are added to dairy products, particularly those labeled as fat-free. Check the label, see what the serving size is and how many grams of sugar is in a serving. Remember that 4 grams of sugar is a teaspoonful, so visualize teaspoons of sugar in the food you buy.
- A component of cheese is particularly addicting, and many people struggle with this.

If you want optimal health, avoid dairy products. Almond, organic soy, and other non-dairy milk are fine, but always buy unsweetened. Products such as non-dairy yogurt and sour cream are available, but watch for sugar, salt, and other unhealthy additives. For additional information, read Dr. Greger's book *How Not to Die*, or go to his website *nutritionfacts.org*.

"Dieting by portion control
doesn't work because one is constantly
fighting addictive drives."

– Joel Fuhrman, M.D.

EGGS: HEALTHY OR NOT?

The purpose of a hen's egg is to provide the nutrients necessary to develop a baby chick. Eggs are packed with protein, fat, cholesterol, vitamins, and minerals. However as Dr. John McDougall, one of the giants in plant-based nutrition puts it, "An egg is the richest of all foods, and far too much of a 'good thing' for people." For example a whole egg has 272 mg. of cholesterol, almost the recommended daily allowance.

It's frustrating when one month we're told by the media that food like eggs should be avoided and then the next month we're told they're okay. The reason for these confusing flip-flops is usually that Big Food does its best to sow seeds of doubt about established science when science shows that their product is unhealthy. This is the same tactic used by the tobacco industry a few decades ago. Here's how this works:

- We know that after eating an egg, triglyceride and cholesterol levels go up for several hours, and we think this is when plaque (atherosclerosis a.k.a. "hardening of the arteries") forms.
- The American Egg Board hires research scientists willing to sell their souls and perform a study with a pre-determined outcome, which supports their product.
- The study shows that blood cholesterol in study subjects after an overnight fast are not elevated, and the Egg Board scientists claim that eggs don't raise cholesterol and are therefore healthy. Of course the damaging post-meal elevation is not mentioned.
- Food and science writers are usually not sophisticated enough to figure out what's going on (it's hard enough for physicians to determine whether a study is legitimate).
- Over 90 percent of "scientific" papers on food are now done by industry-sponsored scientists.

Neal Barnard, M.D., founding president of the PCRM (Physician Committee for Responsible Medicine) recently reviewed the health problems linked to eggs. He noted that recent studies with no industry ties show that people who eat eggs have a significantly elevated risk of:

- Strokes
- Heart attacks—especially in diabetics
- Type 2 diabetes
- Prostate cancer—especially the aggressive type that spreads

It's easy to cook without eggs by substituting ground flaxseed or apple sauce.

My favorite source of unbiased, evidence-based information on nutrition is Dr. Michael Greger's book *How Not to Die* and his website *nutritionfacts.org.*

"You cannot buy your health;
you must earn it through healthy living."

– Joel Fuhrman, M.D.

HEALTH CONCERNS ABOUT ADDED OILS

People are always surprised to hear that they should avoid vegetable oil for optimal health. This is probably because the olive oil-containing Mediterranean Diet is often touted as a healthy diet, which it is compared to the S.A.D. (Standard American Diet). However, people on the Mediterranean Diet are still dying from heart attacks and strokes, whereas people on a plant-based, whole (unprocessed) food diet with no salt, sugar, or added oil are not. Furthermore, this diet is the only one shown to reverse heart disease, as proven by Doctors Ornish and Esselstyn. Any health benefits that the Mediterranean diet has are not due to olive oil, but rather to the intake of vegetables, legumes, fruit, nuts, seeds, and whole grains.

Here is why vegetable oil is not healthy:

- A tablespoonful of any oil has 120 calories, and most Americans don't need those extra, concentrated calories.
- Vegetable oil causes inflammation of the endothelium lining our arteries, resulting in atherosclerotic plaque formation and eventually to plaque rupture—the cause of heart attacks and strokes.
- Oils cause our arteries to stiffen and constrict (you want them to be supple and to dilate).
- Oils are processed, and as with other processed foods, most of the nutrients are lost.
- When you eat whole olives the oil is absorbed slowly, but oil from olives and other vegetables is absorbed rapidly and is immediately stored as fat (Dr. Fuhrman, author of *Eat to Live* and other books says "two minutes from lips to hips" when talking about vegetable oil).
- All oils have saturated fat, which causes our liver to make more LDL (bad cholesterol). Canola has the least at 7 percent, olive oil twice as much at 15 percent, and coconut oil the most at 93 percent (the hype on the Internet touting coconut products are put there by people making money selling them).
- When oils reach their smoke point, carcinogens form.
- The omega-6 to omega-3 ratios in our blood should be 1:1 or 2:1 for optimal health. Most Americans have ratios of 10:1 to 30:1 (way too much omega-6

and too little omega-3), primarily due to the added oil in the diet of most Americans. This abnormal ratio contributes to inflammation, depression, heart disease, and diabetes.

- Oil is fat, and people on the S.A.D. are addicted to salt, sugar, and fat.

It's easy to cook without oil. For sautéing, use wine, sherry, soy sauce, water, vegetable broth, or vinegar. If a baking recipe called for oil, substitute unsweetened apple sauce or ground flaxseed. And you don't need butter or margarine on your toast; just use unsweetened apple sauce and sprinkle cinnamon on it.

Of course, you do need some fat for optimal health, and here's the recommended way to get it:

- All plants have healthy, polyunsaturated fat, some more than others.
- For omega-3, eat 2 tablespoons of ground flaxseed every day (I sprinkle it on my hot cereal in the morning).
- To be sure you get enough omega-3 if you don't eat fish, take a daily 250–450 mg. capsule of algae-derived vegan omega-3 available at Vitamin Cottage (the brand Whole Earth and Sea is reasonably-priced), or order it in liquid form from Dr. Fuhrman at *www.DrFuhrman.com*.
- One handful of raw, unsalted nuts a day. All nuts have good and bad fats, and the healthiest ratio of good to bad is found in walnuts, followed by almonds, pecans, and peanuts (peanuts are technically not a nut but nutritionally they are like nuts).

"The reason Americans are overweight is that they don't enjoy their food enough."

– Sofia Loren, Italian movie actress

(Meaning we don't eat mindfully.)

CUTTING BACK ON SALT
COULD SAVE MILLIONS OF LIVES EACH YEAR

Salt is sodium chloride, which is an essential nutrient for humans and animals. It is thought that early humans consumed about 500 to 750 mg. of sodium a day, which they got from the plant-based diet they ate. Then, centuries ago humans discovered that salt could be used to preserve food, and in most "developed" societies people now eat many times more salt than humans were genetically programed to eat. This is unfortunate because too much salt results in the following health problems:

- Hypertension (high blood pressure), which is the main risk factor for strokes and an important one for heart attacks. According to Dr. Greger (*How Not to Die, nutritionfacts.org*), reducing sodium consumption by just 15 percent worldwide would save millions of lives per year.
- Excess salt directly damages and stiffens arteries, independent of its hypertensive effect.
- Kidney damage can also result from too much salt.
- Water retention, leading to swelling and contributing to heart failure.
- Stomach cancer, particularly prevalent in people who eat pickled (salted) vegetables.

How much salt is recommended? The American Heart Association recommends less than 1,500 mg. of sodium a day, although Dr. Fuhrman in *The End of Heart Disease* states that "for maximal disease prevention, sodium levels should probably be less than 1,000 mg./day." The average American, however, consumes 3,500 mg. a day, and 90 percent of Americans eventually suffer from hypertension. Ideal blood pressure is less than 115/75, and in the few remaining societies in the world untouched by the Western diet, blood pressures remain at that level irrespective of age.

Where do we get excess salt? Surprisingly, the salt shaker isn't the primary culprit:

- In kids, the main source of sodium is pizza (cheese in particular is laden with salt).
- For adults between the ages of 20 and 50, the main source is chicken, which when raised commercially is usually injected with salt water to increase the weight/price.
- For adults over age 50, it's bread.

As previously mentioned, Big Food has people hooked on salt, sugar, and fat. So, they tend to add salt to many products, and it's virtually impossible to find a processed food product with no added salt. The Salt Institute and the food companies use the usual tactic of trying to sow seeds of doubt on established science, but as Dr. Tom Frieden, director of the CDC, said in an article in an issue of the *Journal of the American Medical Association,* "There is incontrovertible evidence of a direct, dose-response relationship between sodium and blood pressure."

Are you concerned that your food will taste bland without salt?

- You will miss it for about 10 to 14 days, and then you will lose your taste for it as the taste receptors in your mouth become more sensitive.
- Add other flavorings such as pepper, onions, garlic, tomatoes, sweet peppers, basil, parsley, thyme, celery, lime, chili powder, rosemary, smoked paprika, curry, coriander, and lemon (per Dr. Greger).
- Try potassium chloride instead of salt (sodium chloride), which looks like salt but has a slightly different after-taste until you get used to it. It's available in the salt section of the grocery store, one brand being NoSalt salt (I put this plus nutritional yeast and cinnamon on my popcorn). The only people who shouldn't take potassium are those with chronic kidney disease.

Read food labels at the grocery store and try to buy things with little or no added salt (no problem if you're in the produce section). A good rule of thumb is to buy foods with fewer milligrams of sodium on the label than there are grams in the serving size. So, as Dr. Greger says, "if it's a 100 gram serving size the product should have less than 100 mg. of sodium." Avoiding salt when eating at restaurants can be difficult because they too take advantage of people's addictions (there's a reason why bars serve salty snacks, which make you thirsty). But request a low-salt meal, and avoid the salt shaker.

LET'S NOT SUGARCOAT
THE DANGERS OF SUGAR

One hundred years ago the average American ate 4–5 pounds of sugar a year; now the average per capita consumption is 150 to 170 pounds a year (visualize 30 to 34, five-pound sacks of sugar).

Big Food cares about their bottom line but not your health. They are doing what the tobacco industry did a few decades ago: hiring scientists to figure out how to make their products more addictive. The scientists found that people get hooked on salt, sugar, and fat, and will buy more of whatever products contain these things.

As Dr. Greger (*How Not to Die* book, *nutritionfacts.org* website) puts it: "The food industries bank their billions by manipulating the pleasure centers within your brain, the so-called dopamine reward system … the same reward system that keeps people smoking cigarettes and snorting cocaine." As with addictive drugs, tolerance to sugar, fat, and salt develops and bigger doses are required to obtain the same pleasure.

Sugar gives you calories without any nutrients. *Nutrition Action Health Letter* is published monthly by the Center For Science in the Public Interest, which has no ties to the food or pharmaceutical industries. They point out that consuming refined sugar (versus sugar in whole foods such as fruit) is associated with the following health problems:

- Obesity
- Cardiovascular disease including heart attacks and strokes
- Rise in LDL (bad cholesterol) and triglycerides
- Type 2 diabetes
- Fatty liver disease (present in one out of five adults and one out of ten teens, which can eventually lead to cirrhosis and liver failure—watch the documentary *Supersize Me)*
- Tooth decay
- Toxic hunger (When you consume sugar, your blood sugar rises for an hour. To counteract that your pancreas secretes insulin and during the second hour your blood sugar often drops lower than it would if you were fasting, causing low blood sugar–hypoglycemia–and "toxic hunger.")

Sugar is added to many products including toothpaste and ketchup, but here are the main sources of sugar in the American diet:

- 47 percent from beverages, primarily soda (a can of non-diet soda contains 10 teaspoons of sugar), but also including fruit drinks (basically flavored sugar water) and sport/energy drinks (fine if you're participating in an endurance athletic event but otherwise not).
- 31 percent from sweets and snacks.

What about artificial sweeteners? They are as addictive as actual sugar, and some have been shown to have other health concerns, so they should be avoided. If you insist on using something sweet for baking, Dr. Greger recommends ground dates, which are a whole, relatively unprocessed food and therefore at least have some nutrients. Other options he suggests are black-strap molasses and prune paste.

When you go grocery shopping, check the food label before you buy something, see what the serving size is and see how many grams of sugar is in a serving. Four grams of sugar is a teaspoon, so visualize teaspoons of sugar. For example, one type of Dave's Killer Bread has 5 grams of sugar per serving size (1 slice) and another 1 gram, so you would want to buy the latter. Low sodium Ezekiel bread has none.

Fruit contains sugar (fructose), so is it okay to eat fruit? Avoid fruit drinks (even if you make your own fresh-squeezed orange juice, it has a very high glycemic index, meaning that when you drink it your blood sugar shoots up). Keep intake of dried fruit including raisins to a minimum because dried fruit has concentrated sugar. But in general, consuming sugar in the form of fresh or frozen fruit is not a problem because components of fruit such as fiber delay the absorption of the sugar. Studies of diabetes who ate unlimited fruit showed that their blood sugars were the same as when they were told to avoid fruit.

So, if you want optimal health, avoid sugar in any form, including products such as honey (sugar is sugar), beet sugar, high fructose corn syrup, and "natural organic cane sugar" (would you buy natural, organic lead or arsenic?). After about 10 to 14 days you will lose your addiction to sweet things, and will experience hunger based on need for calories rather than toxic hunger based on food addiction and swings in insulin and blood sugar levels.

AVOID PROCESSED FOOD

In his book *How Not to Die,* Dr. Michael Greger defines unprocessed food as "nothing bad added, nothing good taken away." In *The Omnivore's Dilemma*, Michael Pollan says, "If it came from a plant, eat it. If it was made in a plant, don't."

The history of processing natural brown rice into white rice in the nineteenth century in Africa illustrates the harm done by processing food. Vitamin B-containing bran was removed from the brown rice. As a result, millions of people who were on a rice-based diet died from beriberi, a disease caused by vitamin-B deficiency. The scientist who figured out why these people were dying won a Nobel prize, and subsequently white rice was fortified with vitamins. (Why weren't the Africans simply advised to go back to eating unprocessed—brown—rice?)

Here are some of the health problems associated with consumption of refined food:

- Obesity; hypertension; high cholesterol and triglycerides; diabetes and pre-diabetes; cardiovascular disease (heart attacks and strokes); auto-immune diseases such as multiple sclerosis; inflammatory diseases such as rheumatoid arthritis; dementia, including Alzheimer's; and some cancers are associated with the consumption of processed food. This is partly due to harm done by the processed foods themselves, such as inflammation and disease-promoting gut bacteria. But harm also occurs because of the antioxidant and other health-promoting plant nutrients people miss out on when they substitute processed food for whole plant food.
- A few decades ago we were told that we should eat less saturated fat, present in meat, dairy, and eggs. The food industry, which is typically more interested in their bottom line than our health, started pushing processed carbohydrates and sugar. It turned out that these things were at least as unhealthy as saturated fat.
- Most of the health-promoting nutrients in plants are removed in the refining process.
- Fiber, which is key to optimal health, is destroyed in processing.
- Processed food has a higher glycemic index than whole food, resulting in

DIET—WHAT WE SHOULD AVOID FOR OPTIMAL HEALTH

blood sugar elevations, which cause the pancreas to secrete more insulin. This eventually leads to pre-diabetes and diabetes.

- Partially-hydrogenated vegetable oil is oil that has been processed to improve shelf life. It causes vascular disease resulting in heart attacks and stroke, and as Dr. Neal Barnard says, "It doesn't improve your shelf life."
- Harmful compounds such as salt and sugar are added to foods to make them more addictive; and harmful artificial food coloring to make food more attractive.

When you go to the grocery store, it's often difficult to tell what is really whole food and what is processed because of misleading advertising (e.g. on cereal boxes and bread wrappers). Here are some tips you can use to avoid processed food:

- Do most of your shopping in the produce aisle and fruit section.
- Read food labels, see what the serving size is, and avoid added salt and sugar (four grams of sugar equals one teaspoon).
- Don't buy cereal in a box. It's better to eat cooked cereal, which you can buy in bulk at Vitamin Cottage and Whole Foods. Steel cut oats are the least processed, followed by rolled oats, but avoid instant. Another good choice is multi-grain cereal, such as seven or ten-grain.
- Any food with intense natural color or flavor has lots of healthful nutrients, but avoid added food dyes, which are harmful.
- Don't buy white rice. Black rice is the healthiest (it's intensely colored), followed by red, and then brown.
- In grocery stores there's a lot of misleading advertising on bread and other wrappers and on cereal boxes. When buying items such as pasta, tortillas, and bread, look at the food label and see if the total carbs:fiber ratio is 5:1 or less (i.e. 4:1 is even better). Multiply the fiber number by 5, and if the result is greater than the number for total carbs, that product has lots of whole grains and fiber. Ezekiel Low Sodium bread, kept in the cooler at Whole Foods and Vitamin Cottage (because it doesn't have a lot of preservatives), is particularly healthful.
- Avoid any product with hydrogenated vegetable oil.
- Avoid making your own processed food, such as juicing and smoothies, which convert low glycemic index food into high glycemic index food, and mechanically destroys fiber. We evolved to chew our food.

AVOIDING TOXINS IN YOUR FOOD

It seems obvious that we should avoid toxins. Here's the scope of the problem:

• According to the CDC, essentially 100 percent of people in the U.S. are contaminated with multiple toxins, such as heavy metals, solvents, endocrine-disrupting chemicals, fire retardants, chemicals from plastic, PCBs, and even pesticides such as DDT that have been banned for years but which stick around for decades in our environment.

• Even if you live in a pristine place such as Rocky Mountain National Park, you are bombarded with many of these chemicals via rain and groundwater.

• Infants are born with toxins in their cord blood, which they get from their mother during pregnancy, and in one study 95 percent of infants had cord blood samples positive for DDT. After birth they get more toxins through breast milk; but formula is worse, so for this and many other reasons breast-feeding is best.

• Children are particularly vulnerable to the adverse effects of toxins and a larger percentage have levels of toxins above the danger level than adults do.

• If you are a woman who wants to clean up your diet before getting pregnant, some toxins can disappear within a few months, but others have such a long half-life it would take 100 years to get rid of them.

Here are a few examples of adverse health effects from toxins:

• According to Neal Barnard, M.D., in his book *Power Foods For The Brain*, heavy metals such as mercury, copper, zinc, aluminum, and heme iron (the iron found in meat versus the non-heme iron in plants) are linked to Alzheimer's.

• According to Dr. Greger (*How Not to Die* book, *nutritionfacts.org*), persistent exposure to pesticides, flame retardants, and other toxic chemicals is linked to Parkinson's Disease and to ALS (Lou Gehrig's Disease).

• Endocrine-disrupting industrial toxins in the aquatic food chain affect testosterone levels, genital development in boys, sexual functioning in men and women, memory capacity, sperm count, and bone density.

• According to Dr. Fuhrman in his book *The End of Heart Disease*, toxins such as

mercury increase the risk of hypertension, heart disease, mental disorders, and endocrine diseases.
- Many toxins are carcinogens, increasing the risk of several types of cancer.

Here are the foods that contain toxins:
- In the modern world, it's almost impossible to completely avoid toxins. Even plants have some toxins, but organically-grown plants have less.
- Animals including fish, being higher on the food chain, have much higher toxin levels than plants. As Dr. Greger puts it: "Consider that before she's slaughtered for meat, a dairy cow may eat seventy-five thousand pounds' worth of plants. The chemicals in the plants can get stored in her fat and build up in her body." We call this process bioaccumulation.
- Most DDT comes from meat and fish.
- Hexachlorobenzene, banned nearly 50 years ago but still present in the environment, is found mainly in dairy, meat, and eggs.
- Dioxins are most concentrated in butter, followed by eggs and processed meat. Dr. Greger says a plant-base diet would wipe out 98 percent of dioxin intake.
- Salmon is one of the worst toxin offenders (sorry!), farmed being worse than wild.

In summary, we all should avoid toxins if we want optimal health, and the way to do this is to eat at the bottom of the food chain, namely plants, and buy organic or grow our own garden. If you think this healthy diet might be bland or restrictive, I'd encourage you to find a restaurant specializing in tasty vegan cooking in your area, or try some new vegan recipes on your own.

HOW BIG FOOD MAKES US SICK AND KILLS US

We all know that too many Americans, including young children, are overweight. Many currently have or develop hypertension, high cholesterol, diabetes, and eventually cardiovascular disease and cancer. These maladies are spreading to the rest of the world as we export our lifestyle. Experts say this is the first generation of children in history who aren't going to live longer lives than their parents. Many of us watched the documentary years ago called *Supersize Me,* where the producer decided to eat 3 meals a day at McDonald's for one month and whenever a supersized portion was offered he would eat it. Within 2 weeks he had gained weight and had developed pre-diabetes, hypertension and fatty liver disease. Clearly, typical fast food is not good for us because it contains too much salt, sugar, and fat, too many refined carbohydrates, and too many calories. But the uneducated shopper can run into just as much trouble at the grocery store.

Unhealthy food is the new tobacco. For decades, Big Tobacco lied to us about the health problems caused by smoking, until the evidence became too overwhelming to deny. Big Food is now using their playbook. The Sunday *New York Times Magazine* had a cover article about how Big Food hires scientists to figure out how to make their products more addictive so that we buy more of them and they make bigger profits. One CEO of a major food company finally couldn't live with himself any longer and resigned, noting that not only are food companies making American adults obese and sick, but children as well.

Food companies make people addicted to salt, sugar, and fat—all of which raise dopamine levels in the pleasure center of the brain, the same center that lights up when people use heroin and other narcotics. To the scientists who work for food companies, the ideal food is the Cheeto, which is crunchy, salty, and oily, so 3 addictive ingredients. But because Cheetos seem "light and crunchy in the mouth," people assume they can eat a lot of them with impunity. Food companies are shameless about adding addictive substances to food. For example, why does organic 365 unsweetened soymilk from Whole Foods have 85 mg. of sodium per serving size (1 cup)? Answer: they want to hook you on their product.

The other way scientists sell their souls to food companies is by conducting studies with predetermined outcomes, which show that a product is safe and healthy when it really isn't (there are many ways to manipulate studies and their outcomes).

When you are grocery shopping, read food labels and first see what the serving size is. Then see what the sugar content is and keep in mind that 4 grams is a teaspoon (you can't visualize grams but you can teaspoons). Then see how much salt is in a serving, keeping in mind that the healthy limit of salt is 1,500 grams a day. Look for the total carbs and fiber on the label. Multiply the fiber number by 5 and if the result is greater than the total carbs number, that product has lots of fiber and whole (unprocessed) grains. (Don't be fooled by bread wrappers and cereal boxes that say "whole grains" because they can say that if the amount of whole grains is minimal.) Also, although organic is preferable in anything without a peal (it isn't helpful to spend more money on organic bananas, oranges, or avocados), don't always assume that just because the label says "natural" or "organic" it is necessarily healthy. For example, Amy's frozen vegan burritos would make a light, healthy lunch if each one didn't contain 620 mg. of salt, more than a third of the daily allowance.

Towards the end of the Obama administration, rules were established to make food labels more consumer-friendly, such as making the serving size more understandable (11 chips instead of 1 oz.), and specifying added sugar instead of just total sugar. But the anti-regulation philosophy of the current administration has caused these rules to be delayed, perhaps forever.

To beat Big Food at their own game, when you shop for groceries spend most of your time in the produce aisles, buying vegetables and fruit. After 10 to 14 days, people get over their addiction to salt, sugar, and fat and lose their taste for those things. It's very difficult to find healthy cereal in a box, so consider buying bulk multi-grain cereal or steel cut oatmeal for example. The healthiest bread I have found is low-sodium Ezekiel, kept in the cooler at Whole Foods (because it doesn't have a lot of preservatives). It has zero sugar and salt.

IS UNHEALTHY EATING THE NEW TOBACCO?

Let's look at the history of medical practice and smoking for an answer. In the mid-20th century, evidence gradually accumulated that smoking was unhealthy, causing lung and other cancers, emphysema, and heart attacks and strokes. However, at that time, essentially everyone smoked, doctors and patients alike. It took some 7,000 studies and tens of thousands of preventable deaths over several years before doctors finally "got it." Part of the reason it took so long is that doctors want controlled studies before they really believe something, but controlled studies of smoking would have been unethical once the dangers became apparent. In spite of the lack of controlled studies, doctors finally did get it, because the evidence of harm from smoking became so overwhelming it was impossible to ignore (the tobacco industry did its best to hide negative evidence and came up with new marketing ploys such as "organic tobacco" and "filtered cigarettes with fewer carcinogens"). Now, very few doctors smoke and they counsel their patients who smoke to quit.

We now have a very similar situation with unhealthy eating. The food industry has people hooked on salt, sugar, and fat, and does its best to sow seeds of doubt about settled science, which shows that these things are unhealthy. The evidence has become overwhelming that meat (including chicken), dairy, eggs, oils, refined food, sugar, and salt contribute to many of our health problems: obesity, hypertension, cardiovascular disease, diabetes, inflammatory conditions, autoimmune disease, dementia, and many forms of cancer. However, doctors don't receive training in nutrition in medical school, and they don't learn about it at most medical conferences, which are often sponsored by pharmaceutical companies. And doctors themselves don't yet understand the power of healthy nutrition, which along with exercise is more effective than any pill we have. So most doctors eat the unhealthy S.A.D. (Standard American Diet). Furthermore, doctors (and hospitals) make huge profits by doing procedures such as stents and bypass surgery, but payment for counseling is low. (Kaiser is based on a different system, and benefits financially when patients stay healthy.)

There's an interesting phenomenon in medicine: the advice doctors give their patients is often based on what they do or don't do themselves. If a doctor exercises he or she will advise their patients to exercise, but if they don't they won't. If a doctor is a

DIET—WHAT WE SHOULD AVOID FOR OPTIMAL HEALTH

skier and their OB patient asks if she can ski while pregnant, the doctor will say it's okay; if the doctor does not ski they will tell their OB patient it's too dangerous. Then there's the joke about how doctors determine if someone has an alcohol problem: anyone who drinks more than they do. The point is that if doctors don't eat a healthy diet they won't counsel their patients to do so.

There are signs of hope though. Kim Williams, recent president of the American College of Cardiology, adopted a plant-based lifestyle after evaluating the options a few years ago, saying that he didn't mind dying so much but he didn't want it to be his fault. My wife and I became plant-based after a nurse practitioner recommended that we read the book *The China Study*. Other plant-based physicians that I'm aware of in Colorado are Kim Scheuer, M.D. and Chris Miller, M.D. in Aspen; Laurie Marbas, M.D. who used to practice in Rifle and is now in Grand Junction; internist Dennis Lipton, M.D. in Vail; orthopedist Richard Cunningham, M.D. in Vail; and Andrew Freeman, M.D., who is a cardiologist at National Jewish in Denver. It will take time, but eventually, doctors will "get it" and start eating a healthy diet themselves, and counsel their patients to do the same thing.

"The time may come when not offering this substantially more effective nutritional approach will be considered malpractice."

– Joel Fuhrman, M.D.

98 HEALTH TIPS FROM A FAMILY DOCTOR

WHAT DIET IS THE HEALTHIEST?

There is conflicting information out there about nutrition, but the science is very clear: The healthiest diet is a plant-based, whole (unprocessed) food, with no salt, sugar, or added oil.

During the Korean and Vietnam wars, autopsies on young American soldiers who were killed revealed that the majority of them had significant atherosclerosis (hardening of the arteries, which is what causes heart attacks and strokes), whereas the Korean and Vietnamese soldiers had none. The difference was not genetic, because Korean and Vietnamese Americans have the same health problems the rest of us have. So it was determined that it was differences in diet, with Americans eating an animal-based and the Asians a plant-based diet. In German-occupied Norway during World War 2, the Germans kept all the meat and dairy for themselves and the rate of heart disease in the Norwegians plummeted but rose again after the war ended and they started eating meat and dairy again.

Over 2 decades ago, cardiologist Dean Ornish, M.D., proved that coronary artery disease could be reversed by the plant-based, whole foods diet. Most M.D.s get little training in nutrition in medical school and most cardiologists aren't interested in prevention, but Dr. Ornish is an exception. Then, T. Colin Campbell, PhD, at Cornell, was studying cancer cells in his lab and found that adding blood from human meat-eaters to them made them grow faster, but adding blood from vegans inhibited their growth. Later he was the lead scientist on the China Study, the biggest population study ever done on nutrition, and found that the people in China who were too poor to afford to eat animal proteins weren't overweight; didn't have hypertension or high cholesterol or type 2 diabetes; didn't have heart attacks or strokes; had very little cancer of the breast, colon, and prostate; had fewer inflammatory diseases such as rheumatoid arthritis; had a low incidence of autoimmune diseases such as M.S.; didn't have osteoporosis or kidney stones; and had a much lower rate of dementia, including Alzheimer's.

Then Caldwell Esselstyn, M.D., who was a general surgeon at the Cleveland Clinic several years ago, was operating on young women who came in with breast cancer, and back then the surgery was the very disfiguring radical mastectomy. He decided there must be a way to prevent breast cancer and found through his own research that women

DIET, WHAT WE SHOULD BE EATING & DRINKING DAILY

on a plant-based diet didn't get this disease. He then proved once again that this diet reversed heart disease.

Part of this diet is what you don't eat: meat including chicken, sea food, dairy, eggs, added oil including olive oil, salt, sugar, and processed food. But even more important is what you do eat every day: a variety of vegetables including cruciferous vegetables; legumes such as beans, lentils and chickpeas; fruit (but not fruit juice or smoothies—chewing is important in releasing nutrients from food); and whole (unprocessed) grains.

Plants have millions of antioxidants and cancer-preventing micronutrients that animal products do not have. Whereas an animal-based diet is acidic and causes inflammation, a plant-based diet is alkaline and anti-inflammatory, which is important in disease prevention because inflammation plays a role in many diseases, including cardiovascular disease. The latest scientific information that supports eating a plant-based diet is that the bacterial flora in our gut influences our health in many ways, and while people on an animal-based diet have disease-causing bacterial flora, plant-based eaters have health-promoting bacteria.

It makes sense that a plant-based diet is the healthiest because that's genetically what we're meant to eat. The human genome developed over some 20 million years, as humans slowly evolved from tree-dwelling plant-eaters. Eventually many human tribes became hunter-gatherers, but by then the human genome was fully developed. Also, most hunter-gatherers subsisted primarily on what they gathered rather than hunted. Furthermore, the jaw and GI structure of humans are that of herbivores, not carnivores.

Currently the Paleo Diet is popular, but other than getting the part right about processed food and simple carbs being bad, there is no scientific evidence to support it (see *nutritionfacts.org* for example). The Mediterranean Diet is currently being touted by the medical establishment as a healthy diet, and it certainly is healthier than the S.A.D. (Standard American Diet), but people on it are still dying from heart attacks and strokes whereas people on a plant-based diet aren't.

If anyone tells you that their diet is better than a plant-based diet, ask them if their diet has been proven to reverse heart disease—the answer will be no.

BEANS ARE BENEFICIAL

In his book *How Not to Die*, Dr. Michael Greger (website *nutritionfacts.org*) lists his daily dozen: foods we should be eating every day and why. This health tip is about legumes—beans of all kinds; lentils, chickpeas (garbanzo beans), and split peas. Dr. Greger recommends 3 servings a day, with serving sizes being 1/4 cup of hummus or bean dip; 1/2 cup of cooked beans, split peas, lentils, tofu, or tempe; or 1 cup of fresh peas or sprouted lentils. Hummus is healthier if oil isn't added; you can make your own or buy Rip Esselstyn's Engine 2 Plant Strong hummus at Whole Foods, which has no added oil. Lentil sprouts, which you can grow yourself, have even more nutrients than mature lentils.

According to Dr. Greger, the most comprehensive analysis of diet and cancer ever performed was published in 2007 by the American Institute for Cancer Research. Their recommendation was to eat whole grains and/or legumes with every meal. In Japan, with one of the healthiest populations in the world (this is changing as Western food is introduced), breakfast almost always includes beans in the form of miso soup with tofu. Legume intake is consistently associated with longer life span throughout the world.

Here's why legumes are so good for you:
- All vegetables have protein, but legumes have the most.
- They contain iron, zinc, fiber, folate, and potassium.
- They have phytates and other cancer-fighting nutrients.
- They lower cholesterol.
- They help regulate blood sugar immediately after a meal, and when anything is eaten for several hours later—called the "second meal effect."
- They help with weight loss, particularly belly fat, which causes insulin resistance/pre-diabetes. According to Bale and Doneen in their book *Beat the Heart Attack Gene*, insulin resistance is the driver of 70 percent of cardiovascular disease.

When patients are advised to increase their legume intake, they sometimes express concerns about gas. It is true that for several days after increasing intake of beans and other legumes, more gas occurs, but once you are on a consistent high-legume intake this problem resolves after several days. Edamame (soybeans) are usually tolerated best—shelled, organic, frozen edamame can be found in many grocery stores. Of interest is that if you are totally plant-based, the rotten egg smell of the flatus and stools that meat and dairy eaters experience resolves—for many reasons, one being that animal products are no longer putrefying in the colon. Here's what Kaiser Permanente recommends in their pamphlet "The Plant-Based Diet, a Healthier Way to Eat" to cut down on gas as you start eating more beans: Put the beans in a large pot and cover with 2 inches of water, bring to a boil for 3 minutes, cover and set aside for 1 to 4 hours, then rinse and drain well.

So, eat more beans, and canned beans are just as healthy as home-cooked, as long as it says no added salt on the label. Here's an easy way to get the recommended amount of beans every day: Put a small handful of frozen edamame in your cooked oatmeal in the morning, along with cinnamon, berries, nuts, and flaxseeds. Another option is to put 1/4 or 1/3 of a can of unsalted black beans, or cooked garbanzo beans, on top of a big salad for lunch, with an oil-free dressing such as balsamic vinegar on top.

Frozen edamame make a good snack for kids, and one that most will eat.

"If it came from a plant, eat it.
If it was made in a plant, don't."

– Michael Pollan

THE TRUTH ABOUT SOY
(IT'S GOOD FOR YOU, WITH SOME CAVEATS)

Like other beans, soybeans have even more protein than other plants. They are also loaded with fiber, iron, magnesium, potassium, and zinc. Soy has been shown to help prevent breast cancer, prevent recurrence of breast cancer, and increase survival in women with breast cancer. It has also been shown to lower cholesterol and risk of heart disease. Soy products such as tofu are less apt to cause uncomfortable intestinal gas and bloating than other varieties of beans.

The healthiest way to eat soy is by eating organic soybeans (edamame), which can be found in the frozen section of most grocery stores. If you thaw them out, they make a convenient, tasty, healthy snack for children and adults. Tempeh is a fermented, unprocessed soy patty and another healthy way to eat soy. Miso is another fermented, whole soy food, in the form of a thick paste, and forms the base for miso soup that is part of the traditional Japanese breakfast. Miso is salty, but the anti-hypertensive effects of the miso seem to outweigh the blood pressure-increasing effect of the salt, according to Dr. Greger (*nutritionfacts.org, How Not to Die* book). Another benefit of miso is that it contains probiotic bacteria. Tofu is processed soy, and half of the nutrients are lost in the processing. However, there are so many nutrients to begin with, that tofu is still very nutritious. Soy milk is also processed, but if putting a little unsweetened soymilk on your oatmeal every morning makes the oatmeal taste better, by all means do it.

One of the reasons soy gets a bad rap is that lots of "fake meat" products such as Beyond Chicken Grilled Strips and many veggie burgers are made from soy. In this case the soy is very processed, resulting in loss of most of the nutrients. However, if these products keep you from eating meat, dairy, and chicken, you're still better off. These meat alternatives often have the same texture and taste as meat or chicken, but it's best to break your addiction to these foods and just "get over" the desire to eat them. (I admit I enjoy Tofurky at Thanksgiving, and have to fight off the carnivores in my family who want to share it.)

The other issue with soy is that Monsanto's Roundup Ready soybeans are the number one genetically modified crop. It's not completely clear yet that GMO food itself causes problems in humans (at least GMO food should be labeled though), but according to Dr. Greger, Roundup and other pesticides even in very small concentrations have estrogenic effects in humans, stimulating the growth of estrogen-receptor-positive breast cancer cells. Roundup Ready GMO soy contains these harmful pesticides, whereas organic soybeans and soy products do not. So, when buying soy products you definitely should buy organic.

One of the false beliefs about soy is that because it contains isoflavones, which are weak phytoestrogens (phyto means plant), it must cause breast cancer. According to Dr. Greger and other experts, the opposite is true. There are two types of estrogen receptors in the body, alpha and beta, and the effects of soy phytoestrogens on different tissues depend on the ratio of alpha to beta receptors in those tissues. So, soy lowers breast cancer risk, which is an anti-estrogen effect, while decreasing hot flashes which is a pro-estrogen effect.

Is there such a thing as too much soy? The answer is yes. In the daily dozen section of Dr. Greger's book *How Not to Die*, legumes are listed as one of the foods we should be eating daily. Three servings a day of legumes are recommended, and a serving of soy would be a cup of edamame or 1/2 cup of tofu or tempeh. In Asia, where the breast cancer rate is 1/6th of what it is in the U.S., they eat quantities like that. However, in the U.S. some people eat much larger amounts of soy in the form of tofu, soymilk, and fake meat, and this counteracts the benefits of the soy. It's always better not to eat too much of one thing, because different vegetables have different health-promoting nutrients.

"Genetics loads the gun, lifestyle pulls the trigger."

– Caldwell Esselstyn, M.D.

BERRIES ARE BERRY GOOD FOR YOU

We should be "eating the rainbow," because plant-based foods with intense colors have high levels of antioxidants. Rust is oxidation of metal; a cut apple turns brown because of oxidation (notice that the peel does not turn brown because that's where most of the antioxidants are). Oxidation in our bodies contributes to aging, cardiovascular disease, and to cancer. Berries are intensely colored and therefore have lots of antioxidants. According to Dr. Fuhrman, author of several books including *The End of Heart Disease,* flavonoid pigments in berries "affect pathways leading to changes in gene expression; detoxification; inhibition of cancer cell growth and proliferation; and inhibition of inflammation and other processes related to heart disease."

Here's what Dr. Greger, author of *How Not to Die,* says about some specific berries:

- Goji berries, available in bulk at Vitamin Cottage, have high concentrations of melatonin, the "sleep hormone," so try eating some in the evening. Zeaxanthin, an antioxidant pigment in gogi berries, protects against macular degeneration and may even treat it. Zeaxanthin is fat soluble, so eating nuts or seeds with goji berries helps with absorption of this nutrient.
- Bilberries, blackberries, strawberries, aronia berries, elderberries, black raspberries, and blueberries (especially the smaller "wild" varieties) all have an antioxidant-laden pigment called anthocyanin.
- Tart cherries (included by Dr. Greger under "berries") have strong anti-inflammatory properties, and can be used to prevent and treat gout.
- Cranberries have been shown in the lab to suppress the growth of several types of human cancer cells, due to the pigment anthocyanin. Unsweetened cranberries are tart, so mix them with some other fruit.

Dr. Fuhrman says that blueberries, strawberries, and blackberries have been shown in animal and human studies to slow or reverse age-related cognitive decline.

Dr. Greger's favorite berries are acai berries, barberries, blackberries, blueberries, cherries (sweet or tart), concord grapes, cranberries, goji berries, kumquats, mulberries, raspberries (black or red), and strawberries. He recommends a serving a day, one serving being 1/2 cup of fresh or frozen or 1/4 cup dried. Sprinkle them on your oatmeal in the morning and/or have a large bowl of them for dessert after dinner, maybe with some unsweetened almond milk. Another way of enjoying berries is to simply blend frozen berries and eat them as "ice cream."

In order to avoid insecticides and other toxins, it's always best to buy organic, and due to the high surface area this is particularly important with berries. Often you can find fresh organic berries on sale in the summer at local grocery stores. At other times of the year, you can purchase frozen berries, which have the same nutritional value that fresh ones do.

"A plant-based diet isn't radical.
What's radical is having gastric surgery
for obesity—a lifestyle problem."

- Greg Feinsinger, M.D.

NON-BERRY FRUIT
IS ALSO GOOD FOR YOU

Dr. Greger notes that few Americans eat the amount of fruit recommended by guidelines. He recommends 3 servings a day, with a serving size being 1 medium-sized fruit such as an apple or pear or orange; 1 cup of cut-up fruit; or 1/4 cup of dried fruit. Among his favorite non-berry fruits are apples, dried apricots, cantaloupe, clementines, dates, dried figs, grapefruit, honeydew, kiwifruit, lemons, limes, lychees, mangoes, nectarines, oranges, papaya, passion fruit, peaches, pears, pineapple, plums (especially black ones), pluots, pomegranates, prunes, tangerines, and watermelon.

Here are a few tips about fruit, from Dr. Greger's *How Not to Die*:

- Watermelon has few antioxidants but their seeds have lots, so avoid seedless and eat the seeds.
- Watermelon contains a compound called citrulline that boosts the activity of an enzyme that works like viagra, and yellow watermelon has more of this than red.
- Kiwifruit helps with insomnia, the dose being two, one hour before bedtime. It also boosts immune function. Rarely people are allergic to Kiwifruit.
- Citrus helps with DNA repair. Certain citrus compounds concentrate in breast tissue and help prevent breast cancer, and there are more of these in the peel. So, eat an orange or half a grapefruit every morning as part of your breakfast, and include some orange peel. You can grate your own peel but if you do, be sure to buy organic and wash the fruit before grating. Another option is to buy a bag of organic, grated orange peel at Vitamin Cottage.
- Grapefruit can affect the metabolism of certain pharmaceuticals such as some statins. So, if you're taking a statin, check with your provider or pharmacist to see if you need to limit your intake of grapefruit.

People often wonder if they should limit fruit because of the sugar it contains. Someone asked Dr. Greger this question after his talk at the Colorado Veg Fest in Denver, Colorado, and he said that the only way you're going to hurt yourself with fruit is if you drop a 20-pound watermelon on your foot. Sugar from eating whole fruit is not

DIET, WHAT WE SHOULD BE EATING & DRINKING DAILY

harmful, but avoid fruit juices, which are essentially flavored sugar water. Even if you make your own orange juice, your blood sugar rises sharply when you drink it, which leads to many problems such as diabetes and cardiovascular disease. This does not occur if you eat an orange. For this and other reasons, it is best to chew your fruit rather than drink it by juicing or making a smoothie.

"If beef is your idea of 'real food for real people,'
you'd better live real close to a real good hospital."

– Neal Barnard, M.D.

CRUCIFEROUS VEGETABLES ROCK

Cruciferous vegetables have four-petaled flowers, suggestive of a cross, and the name comes from *crux*, the Latin word for cross. This family of vegetables includes kale, cabbage, arugula, bok choy, broccoli, cauliflower, brussels sprouts, collard greens, horseradish, mustard greens, radishes, turnip greens, and water cress. In his book *How Not to Die* Dr. Michael Greger (*nutritionfacts.org*) recommends one serving of cruciferous vegetables a day, serving sizes being 1/2 cup of chopped, 1/4 cup of sprouts, or one tablespoon of horseradish.

The reason cruciferous vegetables are so good for you is that they (especially broccoli and kale, which have been studied the most) have been shown to:
- Prevent propagation of cancer cells in a petre dish in the lab
- Target breast cancer stem cells
- Reduce the risk of prostate cancer progression
- Prevent DNA damage and metastatic cancer spread
- Help fight infections
- Help protect us from environmental pollutants
- Decrease inflammation
- Decrease oxidation and thereby help prevent cardiovascular disease
- Protect our brain and eyesight, reduce nasal allergy inflammation, manage type 2 diabetes

Here's something you need to know about eating cruciferous vegetables: Sulforaphane is one of the of the most health-promoting chemicals in cruciferous vegetables. It comes from a precursor compound and in order to be converted into sulforaphane an enzyme called myrosinase is required, which is destroyed by heat. To obtain the health benefits of sulforaphane, your options are:
- Eat your cruciferous vegetables raw, as in salads, and chew well to enable the myrosinase to do its work.
- Eat some raw cruciferous vegetables just before you eat cooked ones, so myrosinase is available.
- Chop up the vegetables into small pieces and wait 40 minutes before cooking, so the myrosinase has time to convert the precursor to sulforaphane.

- If you are making a smoothie, use raw rather than cooked cruciferous veggies or blend and wait forty minutes before making soup.
- Sprinkle mustard powder or add Daikon, regular radishes, horseradish, or wasabi to cooked cruciferous veggies to supply the myrosinase.
- Commercially-produced cruciferous veggies are flash-cooked before freezing, which destroys the myrosinase, so if you want to get the health benefits of the sulforaphane you have to add the mustard or radish after thawing out the frozen veggies.

"Since the foods Americans consume are so calorie-rich,
we have all been trying to diet by eating smaller portions of low-nutrient foods.
We not only have to suffer hunger but also wind up with perverted cravings
because we are nutrient-deficient to boot."

- Joel Fuhrman, M.D.

GREENS ARE GOOD FOR YOU

According to Dr. Michael Greger's book *How Not to Die*, if you want optimal health, it is imperative to eat a variety of greens every day. As a matter of fact, Dr. Greger says that greens have the most nutrients per calorie of any food. His favorites greens are arugula, beet greens, collard greens, kale, mesclun mix (assorted young salad greens), mustard greens, sorrel, spinach, Swiss chard, and turnip greens. Some of these are covered in the health tip on cruciferous vegetables: arugula, kale, mustard and turnip greens, cabbage, and others.

Intense color in fruits and vegetables is associated with a particularly high level of health-promoting nutrients such as antioxidants. We should "eat the rainbow" every day. The green in greens is chlorophyll, and chlorophyll itself reverses DNA damage in lab and human studies, thereby helping to prevent cancer. But there are other colors in greens as well, masked by the chlorophyll (like the colors of fall leaves which become apparent only after the green chlorophyll dissipates). In addition to cancer prevention, greens offer protection against other diseases, including a 20 percent reduction in risk for heart attacks and strokes for every additional daily serving.

Dr. Greger recommends 2 servings of greens a day, a serving being 1 cup of raw or 1/2 cup of cooked. Sprouted greens have even more nutrients than the mature vegetable. Dr. Greger does not recommend alfalfa sprouts however, because of 28 cases of Salmonella food poisoning linked to this food over the past 12 years (to put this in perspective, there are some 142,000 cases a year of Salmonella food poisoning from eggs).

What about greens for people on Coumadin (warfarin)—used for anti-coagulation? One of the many nutrients that greens contain is vitamin K, which reverses the effect of Coumadin. The problem arises when someone is stable on a particular Coumadin dose and then suddenly eats a lot of greens. It's unfortunate that many providers tell their patients on Coumadin to avoid greens, which Dr. Greger calls "the healthiest food on the planet." I tell patients on Coumadin to eat greens every day without fail, but about the same amount every day. The Coumadin dose then needs to be increased (do not try this own your own without checking with your provider). Another strategy for people needing a "blood thinner" is to put them on one that is not affected by intake of vitamin K, such as Pradaxa.

Many of the nutrients in greens are absorbed better with a small amount of fat. Another health tip discusses the problems with oil (even olive oil), so avoid dressings with oil. Instead, use fat-free dressing such as balsamic vinegar, but add a few olives, a small amount of avocado, nuts and/or seeds to your salad. A tasty dressing from TrueNorth Health Center in Santa Rosa, California, is to blend:

2 tablespoons almond meal
3 cloves crushed garlic
3 tablespoons Dijon mustard
3 tablespoons nutritional yeast flakes
2 tablespoons white miso
3 tablespoons lemon juice
1/3 cup of water

So, your mother was right when she said "eat your greens."

"The fat you eat is the fat you wear."

– John A. McDougall, M.D.

DIET, WHAT WE SHOULD BE EATING & DRINKING DAILY

OTHER VEGETABLES

In the previous health tip, I reviewed greens, which Dr. Greger calls the food with the most nutrients per calorie. However, different plants offer different benefits, so we should be eating a variety every day, and "other vegetables" follows greens in his daily dozen list.

Dr. Greger's favorite "other vegetables" are artichokes, asparagus, beets, bell peppers, carrots, corn, garlic, mushrooms, okra, onions, purple potatoes, pumpkin, squash, sweet potatoes/yams, tomatoes, zucchini, and sea vegetables (e.g. seaweed used in sushi, miso soup, and other Japanese delicacies). He recommends eating 2 servings of some of these daily, a serving being 1 cup of raw leafy vegetables, 1/2 cup raw or cooked non-leafy vegetables, 1/2 cup of vegetable juice, or 1/4 cup of dried mushrooms.

I have written before about the importance of "eating the rainbow," because intense color (and flavor) is associated with a high level of antioxidants and other plant nutrients. Mushrooms are an exception because they are not colorful, but in spite of that, they have a high level of an antioxidant called ergothioneine, one of the few that get inside of mitochondria (the microscopic power plants within your cells, where DNA is especially vulnerable to free-radical/oxidative damage). The caution with mushrooms, especially morels, is that they contain a toxin which is destroyed by cooking. It's best not to eat mushrooms raw.

Sweet potatoes (yams) are intensely colored and are a super food—one of the healthiest things you can eat, especially if you include the skin, which has even more antioxidant power than the orange part. They are also one of the foods with the best nutrients per dollar ratio. White potatoes are much less healthy, so buy purple or blue potatoes instead.

A study published in the journal *Food Chemistry* pitted 34 common vegetables in the lab against 8 different types of human cancer cells. They found that breast cancer cells stopped growing when cauliflower, brussels sprouts, green onions, leeks, and garlic were added. Radishes were 100 percent effective in halting growth of stomach cancer but were not effective against pancreatic cancer. Orange bell peppers were useless against stomach cancer but suppressed prostate cancer cell growth by 75 percent. The take home message according to the researchers was "a diversified diet, containing several distinct classes of vegetables is essential for effective prevention of cancer." In particular, cruciferous vegetables and Allium vegetables (garlic, leeks and onions) are important.

What's the best way to cook vegetables? Deep-fried foods of any kind have been associated with higher cancer risk per Dr. Greger. Deep frying vegetables causes formation of the carcinogen acrylamide (with meat, including chicken, deep frying causes carcinogens called heterocyclic amines). Dr. Greger points out that "the excess lifetime cancer risk attributable to the consumption of french fries in young children may be as high as one or two in ten thousand—meaning about 1 in 10,000 boys and girls eating french fries may develop cancer" that they otherwise would not have gotten.

The most antioxidant loss occurs when vegetables are boiled and pressure-cooked—griddling (cooking in a thick frying pan with no oil) and microwaving resulted in the least. Bell peppers are best eaten raw. Artichokes, beets, and onions, carrots, and celery are resistant to antioxidant loss no matter how you cook them. Cooking tomatoes and green beans releases nutrients when cooked by any method except boiling, that you don't get eating them raw.

The bottom line is eat large portions of a variety of vegetables every day for optimal health, and don't get too hung up on whether to eat them raw or cooked, and how to cook them, as long as you don't fry them.

"The art of medicine consists in amusing the patient
while nature cures the disease."

– Voltaire, French Enlightenment philosopher

(Your body has an amazing ability to heal itself
if you give it the right tools: exercise and healthy food.)

NUTS ABOUT NUTS (AND SEEDS)

Nuts and seeds are part of Dr. Greger's daily dozen, foods we should be eating every day (Michael Greger, M.D. is the author of *How Not to Die* and has the website *nutritionfacts.org*). Technically nuts are seeds, and are therefore full of micronutrients. He points out that there are multiple studies showing that people who eat nuts tend to live longer and suffer fewer deaths from cancer, heart disease, and respiratory disease. His favorite nuts are walnuts, pecans, almonds, Brazil nuts, cashews, hazelnuts, macadamia nuts, pistachios, and peanuts (peanuts are technically legumes like beans but nutritionally are like nuts). Walnuts are the healthiest nut due to their high antioxidant and omega-3 level, and their ability to suppress cancer cell growth.

We should all eat a handful of walnuts a day for brain and cardiovascular health among other reasons. If walnuts are pricey, almonds, pecans, and peanuts are next best. The nuts you eat should be unsalted, because Americans eat too much salt, which leads to hypertension. Also, don't buy toasted nuts, mainly because if they taste too good you will eat more than a handful.

Some patients are concerned about nuts being high in calories. However, studies show that people who eat nuts don't gain the weight you would expect based on the calories. This appears to be due to satiation after eating a handful of nuts, which keeps you from eating too much of other, less healthy food; failure to absorb some of the fat; and increased fat-burning metabolism. Nuts can also be used as healthy sources of fat to make rich, creamy sauces or salad dressings.

What about nut butter? One fourth cup of nuts equals two tablespoons of nut butter, so that would be your serving of nuts for the day. Be sure the nut butter has nothing but nuts on the list of ingredients, and that it has not been processed, which causes harmful trans-fats.

Dr. Greger's favorite seeds are flaxseeds, followed by chia, pumpkin, sesame, and sunflower seeds. Because they don't eat fish, people on a plant-based diet need to get omega-3 from other sources: two tablespoons of ground flaxseed a day are an important source of healthy fats for plant-based people. Flaxseeds have also been shown to reduce high blood pressure, and because of phytonutrients called lignans help prevent breast and prostate cancer. You can also use ground flaxseeds in recipes as an egg or oil replacement.

DIET, WHAT WE SHOULD BE EATING & DRINKING DAILY

Another way of getting healthy fats is to sprinkle unsalted pumpkin and sunflower seeds on your salads, which help you absorb the fat-soluble vitamins in your greens.

Your body converts flaxseeds and nuts to omega-3, which is important for brain health. For genetic reasons, some people might not convert enough, so if you are totally vegan and don't eat fish, consider also taking a 250–450 mg. supplement of vegan, algae-derived omega-3 daily to be on the safe side.

"Even after years of beating yourself up with a horrible diet, your body can reverse the damage, open back up the arteries— even reverse the progression of some cancers. Amazing!"

– Michael Greger, M.D.

TURMERIC, THE WONDER SPICE

India has one of the lowest rates of cancer in the world, and it's thought that turmeric, which makes curry yellow, is the reason. Inflammation and oxidation contribute to several diseases, including cancer. We know that plants with intense flavor (e.g. herbs and spices) and color have an abundance of antioxidants, and many of these plants also have anti-inflammatory effects. Turmeric has both intense color and intense flavor.

Current technology allows scientists to detect DNA damage. Turmeric has been shown in the lab to prevent and reverse DNA damage. It also prevents and reverses DNA damage in living humans, as in the following two studies: (1) A study of radiology technicians, who were exposed to DNA-damaging radiation, showed less damage if they took daily turmeric. (2) Smoking causes DNA damage, which is prevented if smokers take daily turmeric. Prevention and repair of DNA damage is no doubt one of the reasons turmeric helps prevent cancer.

Multiple studies have been done on turmeric since the turn of the century, as outlined in Dr. Greger's well-referenced book *How Not to Die* and his website *nutritionfacts.org.* Here are some of the conditions that turmeric has been shown to help:

- Turmeric has been shown in the lab to kill many kinds of cancer cells, including colon, breast, brain, lung, pancreas, and multiple myeloma (a blood cancer), although that doesn't necessarily mean it reverses cancer in living human beings.
- Turmeric blocks pre-cancerous mutations in lungs of smokers and if lung cancer is already present, turmeric helps prevent it from growing and spreading.
- Turmeric taken orally gets rid of pre-cancerous cell clusters in the colon. In patients who already have advanced colon cancer, turmeric has been shown in some cases to stop the growth of chemotherapy and radiation-resistant tumors.
- When applied directly to cancer, turmeric reverses cancer of the mouth, stomach, colon, bladder, cervix, skin, vulva, and breast (breast cancer unresponsive to chemo and radiation that has extended through the skin).
- Arsenic is a carcinogenic heavy metal, thought to cause cancer by creating free radicals (i.e. oxidation). Turmeric helps prevent this DNA damage in people exposed to arsenic and also chelates (binds to) arsenic.
- In India, turmeric drops are used to treat conjunctivitis (pink eye). It is as effec-

tive as steroids against a more serious eye inflammation called uveitis, but without the side effects of steroids. It's even effective in treating the most severe type of eye inflammation called orbital pseudotumor.

- Insulin resistance, where muscles and organs are unable to use insulin like they should, leads to pre-diabetes and type 2 diabetes. Turmeric improves insulin sensitivity, preventing pre-diabetes from progressing to diabetes. It also improves blood sugar and A1C levels in people who already have type 2 diabetes.

- People given daily turmeric prior to and following surgery have less postoperative pain and fatigue.

- A delicate organ system called the endothelium lines our arteries. Endothelial dysfunction, caused by oxidation and inflammation, contributes to high blood pressure and cardiovascular disease, eventually leading to heart attacks and stroke. Turmeric helps endothelial dysfunction. (Interestingly, India has a high rate of heart disease in spite of turmeric in their diet—due to processed butter called ghee used in Indian cooking.)

- Turmeric has been shown to help prevent Alzheimer's disease and to improve symptoms in people who already have it (Alzheimer's is probably an inflammatory and vascular disease).

- It can reverse rheumatoid arthritis and treat symptoms of degenerative arthritis.

- It has been shown to be effective against ulcerative colitis—an inflammatory condition.

- Turmeric can heal kidney damage in people with Lupus—an autoimmune/inflammatory condition.

Some of the studies on turmeric looked at a component of turmeric called curcumin. Supplement and pharmaceutical companies are always trying to find the "silver bullet" in natural foods, so they can patent and sell it. However, for many conditions curcumin is less effective than turmeric, which has many additional healthful micronutrients. So, it's best to use the whole food—in this case turmeric.

The second half of Dr. Greger's book is about what we should be eating every day, and he has his daily dozen, one of which is herbs and spices. He recommends 1/4 teaspoon of ground turmeric a day, which is about the daily amount in the diet of most people in India. Powdered turmeric can be purchased in bulk at Vitamin Cottage, and 1/4 teaspoon is equivalent to about 1/4 inches of grated turmeric root. You can stir the powder or grated root into a small amount of kombucha or juice, or put it on something like your cereal. The study on Alzheimer's used a whole teaspoon—more than that may cause instead of prevent damage. Adding black pepper to Turmeric increases the blood level by 2,000 percent, so that is not recommend. Cooked turmeric is best for DNA repair, and raw turmeric for inflammation.

OTHER BENEFICIAL SPICES

As discussed in previous health tips, many herbs and spices used for centuries in various cultures as "folk medicine" have been studied in recent years, and some have been found to be effective and others haven't. This health tip is about other herbs and spices that have proven to be effective, based on Dr. Greger's book *How Not to Die*.

- Fenugreek, used in Indian and Middle Eastern cooking, has been shown to improve weight-lifting power. One study showed that athletes could leg press an extra 80 pounds when taking fenugreek, compared to a placebo group.
- Cilantro is used for its flavor in Mexican, Southeast Asian, and other cultures. A study of arthritis sufferers showed that their pain and inflammation was reduced compared to a placebo after taking about 20 sprigs of cilantro a day for 2 months. It also lowers uric acid levels and therefore might be useful in preventing and treating gout.
- Cayenne pepper contains capsaicin, which causes a burning sensation when it comes in contact with skin and mucous membranes. When used repetitively on painful areas, it desensitizes the pain fibers, causing pain to diminish and even resolve. Capsaicin has been used successfully for several pain syndromes, including post-shingles pain and cluster headaches. Although it seems counter-intuitive, after several days coated capsules of red pepper powder decreased abdominal pain in people who suffer from IBS (irritable bowel syndrome) and chronic indigestion (dyspepsia).
- Oregano has been shown in the lab to reduce DNA damage caused by radiation. Other lab experiments show that it has anticancer and anti-inflammatory properties. Marjoram, a closely-related herb inhibited breast cancer cells in the lab. The only study done on live people showed that after a month daily marjoram tea reduced abnormally high hormone levels in PCOS (polycystic ovarian syndrome) sufferers.
- Cinnamon: There are 2 types—cassia (a.k.a. Chinese cinnamon) and Ceylon cinnamon. If the label just says "cinnamon," it is usually cassia, which contains coumarin. This compound can cause liver toxicity, so daily intake of cinnamon should be kept at well under one teaspoon a day, and much less for children.

Ceylon cinnamon doesn't contain coumarin, but may not have the health benefits of cassia cinnamon, which brings down blood sugars in diabetes as well as the common diabetic drug metformin does (and without the side effects).

- Amla is also known as dried Indian gooseberry fruit, and is often used in traditional Indian Ayurvedic medicine. Amla has a very high antioxidant content, which probably translates into many health benefits, but studies have yet to be done.
- Poppy seeds contain some natural morphine and codeine and have been used for pain in European folk medicine. High doses can cause positive drug screens and can cause respiratory depression—in one case an infant given poppy seeds stopped breathing.
- Dr. Greger's favorite spice mixes are "pumpkin pie spice, curry powder, chili powder, Chinese five-spice powder, an Indian spice blend called garam masala, an Ethiopian blend called berbere, Italian seasoning, poultry seasoning, and Middle Eastern blend called za'atar." These spice blends likely have synergistic medicinal benefits, but studies haven't been done yet.

It needs to be stressed that doses of these spices that have been proven to promote health were relatively small when used in traditional folk medicine—a pinch of this and a pinch of that. If a little is good doesn't mean that a lot is better, and high doses of these things can be harmful.

"We should all be eating
fruits and vegetables as if our lives depend on it
—because they do."

- Michael Greger, M.D.

DIET, WHAT WE SHOULD BE EATING & DRINKING DAILY

WHOLE GRAINS ARE GOOD FOR YOU

A few decades ago when Americans were becoming more obese, we were told we needed to eat less fat. The food industry took advantage of this and started offering us food with "low-fat" and "no fat." Unfortunately, these products contained sugar and refined grains, were just as addictive as foods with fat, and were just as unhealthy—and our obesity epidemic worsened.

Then, we were told we were eating too many processed, simple carbs, and people were led to believe that all carbs were bad. The truth is that there are good fats (plant fats) and bad (saturated and trans from animal products). And there are also good carbs (whole, unrefined) and bad carbs (processed, sugary).

Whole grains contain complex carbohydrates, protein, healthy polyunsaturated fat, antioxidants, and other health-promoting nutrients. There are some diets out there that advise against eating grains, but this advice is not based on good science. For example, there are claims that grains cause inflammation, but well-done studies show that whole grains actually prevent and decrease inflammation. Many studies, including Harvard's Nurses' Health Study, show that people who eat whole grains daily live longer and reduce their risk of heart disease, type 2 diabetes, obesity and strokes.

Many health professionals including some dietitians and diabetic educators still adhere to the old dictum that diabetics should avoid any type of carbohydrate. Certainly diabetics, like the rest of us, should avoid processed carbs, but current nutrition science tells us that diabetics do fine with, and even benefit from, unprocessed carbs (for example see John McDougall's book *The Starch Solution*).

As with any type of food, when grains are processed, fiber and most of the nutrients are removed. Processing also changes grains from a low glycemic food (blood sugar remains stable) into a high glycemic index food (blood sugar shoots up). When blood sugar increases, the pancreas secretes more insulin, which leads to obesity, diabetes, and cardiovascular disease.

As previously mentioned, intense color is associated with an abundance of plant micro-nutrients. The healthiest rice is black rice, second is red, third brown, and you should avoid white rice. In regard to bread, Dr. Fuhrman—author of many books including *Eat to Live*—says "the whiter your bread the sooner you're dead." The healthiest tortillas are dark, multi-grain varieties followed by corn tortillas (be sure there is no lard in them). Whole and multi-grain pasta tastes much better than they used to, and Dr. Greger's favorite brand is Bionaturae. You will find whole grain pasta much more satiating than white pasta, so you won't eat as much.

In the grocery store, you will find misleading advertising on wrappers and cereal boxes. Food companies can say a product has "whole grains" even if the amount is minimal. So, look at the food label, see what the total carbs number is and then the number for grams of fiber. The ratio of total carbs:fiber should be 5:1 or less. Multiply the grams of fiber by 5, and if that number is greater than the number for total carbs, that product has lots of whole grains and fiber. You can use this formula for cold cereal (best not to buy cold cereal though, due to added salt, sugar, and oil), and for pasta, tortillas, and bread.

Oats deserve special mention, because they contain unique anti-inflammatory compounds called avenanthramides. For decades oatmeal baths have been used for skin inflammation, and oatmeal lotion relieves skin itching and irritation. Eating oatmeal reduces inflammation in our bodies. The least processed form of oats is steel cut oats, available in bulk at many grocery stores. Rolled oats are next best, but avoid instant oats. Another healthy hot cereal is multi-grain.

Dr. Greger's favorite whole grains are barley, unprocessed rice, buckwheat, millet, oats, popcorn (try nutritional yeast, cinnamon, and NoSalt salt on it), quinoa, rye, teff, whole-wheat pasta, and wild rice. Three servings of whole grains a day are recommended, a serving being 1/2 cup of hot cereal or cooked grains or pasta or corn kernels; 1 cup of cold cereal; 1 tortilla or slice of bread; or 3 cups of popped popcorn.

What about gluten in wheat? Some people have celiac disease, which can be very serious, and they must avoid any wheat products. There are other people who seem to have "gluten sensitivity" and if they feel better avoiding gluten they should do it. But for the rest of us, eating gluten/wheat is fine, as long as it's unprocessed.

WHAT TO DRINK?

Adequate fluid intake is clearly important for optimal health. Dehydration leads to concentrated urine and "thicker" blood, and if severe enough can lead to death. Studies have shown a 50 percent decrease in bladder cancer and heart disease in people who drink 8 or more cups of water a day. Dr. Greger recommends 5 or more glasses of tap water a day—tap instead of bottled because it is less expensive, has less environmental impact, and often has less chemical and microbial contamination.

Like anything, there can be too much of a good thing, and some people over-hydrate. If you are a couch potato you obviously don't need to drink as much water as someone who has a physical job or who sweats while exercising. What I tell patients is to drink enough so they are urinating every hour or so throughout the day, and their urine should be clear to pale yellow. If their urine is dark yellow, they are under-hydrated (a caveat is that B-vitamin pills make your urine dark yellow for several hours). To make water less boring, try adding carbonation, lemon, lime, or mint.

An issue of *Nutrition Action Health Letter* notes that "America's drinking water is in trouble." Most Americans no longer have to worry about getting parasitic, bacterial, or viral illnesses from water, but we now have to worry about industrial, pharmaceutical, and other chemical contaminants, as well as naturally occurring ones such as arsenic and lead (think Flint, Michigan). If you have an old house that could possibly have lead pipes, get your water tested by going to: Safe Drinking Water Hotline or *epa.gov/dwlabcert* and click on contact information for certification programs and then certified laboratories. If you want to see what's in your town's water, check your Consumer Confidence Report: *epa.gov/ccr* or call EPA's Safe Drinking Water Hotline at 800-426-4791. In any case, we all should consider using a filter for our drinking water, and the website to check out different filters is *nsf.org*.

What about other fluids?

- Fruit and non-starchy vegetables have a high water content, which counts as part of your daily fluid requirement (I find that I need to drink less since going plant-based several years ago).
- Tea has many health-promoting micronutrients. According to Dr. Greger, a combination of berry and hibiscus has the most, with green tea close behind.

DIET, WHAT WE SHOULD BE EATING & DRINKING DAILY

It's best to buy loose-leaf tea rather than bags, and it should be organic. You can find such tea on the Internet and at tea-specialty shops. You can make hot tea or cold-steep it.

- Coffee has some health benefits, but not as many as tea. Over the years I have seen many patients with GERD (acid reflux), which went away after completely stopping coffee (even decaf has some caffeine).
- Alcohol is not recommended as a source of fluids, because other than beer it is dehydrating. And any alcohol other than small amounts of red wine increases risk of breast cancer in women.
- The Beverage Guidance Panel ranked milk far down the list of recommended beverages due to links with prostate and ovarian cancer.
- Soda is not recommended in any form or quantity. Sugar is an issue with regular soda (10 teaspoons in a can) and there are other health issues with sugar-free soda.
- Sports drinks such as Gatorade are not healthy unless you are exercising vigorously, because of their high sugar, salt, and calorie content.
- Avoid fruit juices, which are basically flavored sugar water.

"Most brown bread is merely white bread with a fake tan."

– Joel Fuhrman, M.D.

WHY FIBER IS SO FABULOUS

There is a severe fiber deficiency in America, the land of plenty. Only three percent of us eat the minimum 32 grams of fiber a day recommended by U.S. guidelines. Dr. Michael Greger, M.D. notes in his book *How Not to Die* and his website *nutritionfacts.org* that, based on analysis of fossilized stool (he calls this "Paleopoop") and the diets of primitive cultures existing today, we evolved over millions of years eating 100 grams or more of fiber a day. Ideally, we still should do that.

There are two types of fiber. Soluble fiber means it is soluble in water, and examples are oats (the gelatinous substance when you cook oatmeal), peas, beans, apples, citrus, carrots, and barley. Foods with insoluble fiber include whole grains, wheat bran, nuts, beans, cauliflower, and potatoes eaten with the skin.

A large portion of insoluble fiber-containing foods are digested, but the insoluble part of them goes right through the GI tract, undigested—but insoluble fiber feeds the health-promoting bacteria in our gut microbiome. Animals have bones that hold them up and plants have fiber. Meat, dairy, and other animal products do not contain fiber, but all unprocessed plant products do. We know that people who eat lots of fiber have a lower incidence of several diseases, but it's difficult to tell in studies whether these health benefits are from the fiber, from the increased consumption of plant products, or from decrease in consumption of animal products. However, Dr. Greger, Dr. Fuhrman, Dr. Ornish, and other nutrition experts describe well-done studies that show that eating more fiber offers the following benefits:

- Fiber has no calories, yet due to its bulk it fills people up, thereby preventing and reversing obesity.
- It lowers blood pressure.
- It lowers cholesterol.
- It prevents insulin spikes and helps prevent and reverse pre-diabetes and type 2 diabetes.
- It decreases strokes and heart attacks.
- It treats and prevents constipation by increasing stool bulk and transit time (the time it takes for stool to go through the GI tract).
- By decreasing straining to have a stool, fiber decreases the incidence of hiatal

DIET, WHAT WE SHOULD BE EATING & DRINKING DAILY

hernia, GERD (acid reflux), hemorrhoids, hernias, and diverticulosis (small pouches off the wall of the colon that can lead to diverticulitis).

• It decreases the incidence of breast and colon cancer.

• Fiber binds toxins such as heavy metals, and removes them in your stool.

How do you increase your intake of fiber? Basically, decrease or avoid animal products and eat fruit, whole (unprocessed) grains, and a variety of vegetables including legumes. In general, you want to buy your food in the produce section of the grocery store. When you do buy something in a box or wrapper (e.g. bread) check the food label for the serving size and then fiber per serving. If the total carb:fiber ratio is 5:1 or less, the product has lots of fiber and whole grains (multiply the fiber number by 5 and that number should be greater than the number for total carbs). Here are fiber contents of some foods that don't come in a wrapper or box:

• Black beans, 1 cup: 19 grams of fiber.

• Cooked broccoli, 3/4 cup: 7 gm.

• Oatmeal, 3/4 cup: 7.7 gm.

• Garbanzo beans, 1 cup: 12 gm.

• Three dried figs: 10.5 gm.

• Swiss chard cooked, 1/2 cup: 4 gm.

• One pear: 4 gm.

• Raspberries, 1/2 cup: 4.6 gm.

• One yam with the skin: 6.8 gm.

How about taking fiber supplements such as Metamucil or Benefiber? As is always the case, the pharmaceutical industry cannot compete with Mother Nature. There have been a few studies that questioned some of the above benefits of fiber, but for the most part they were done with fiber supplements (in some cases natural fiber was used but in amounts far below ideal). There is no substitute for increasing fiber-containing foods in your diet.

RUMINATIONS ON WHAT'S RADICAL AND RESTRICTIVE

Occasionally, someone will question whether a plant-based diet is too radical or restrictive.

Let's address the radical issue first:

- Until recently, when we started exporting the S.A.D. (Standard American Diet) to the rest of the world, the majority of people on the planet were on a plant-based diet, so historically it's not radical.
- Caldwell Esselstyn, M.D., of the Cleveland Clinic and cardiologist Dean Ornish, M.D., in California proved years ago using sequential arteriograms that this diet reverses heart disease. Dr. Esselstyn says that what should be considered radical is going in the hospital, having your chest cut open and the blockages in your arteries bypassed, risking serious complications including death, and incurring tens of thousands of dollars in medical expenses.
- Plant-based nutrition has no side effects, costs nothing, and treats and reverses the cause of heart disease (atherosclerosis a.k.a. hardening of the arteries), extends life and within days improves quality of life (e.g. angina resolves). So maybe it's radical that primary care doctors and cardiologists fail to talk to their patients about the plant-based option before they recommend stents or bypass surgery, especially given that these procedures have never been shown to prolong life (except in the setting of an acute heart attack) or improve quality of life.
- Maybe what's radical is to undergo costly and potentially dangerous obesity surgery such as stomach stapling or banding, when lifestyle modification is a cure.
- Type 2 diabetes is preventable and reversible with plant-based nutrition. Maybe it's radical that weight-loss surgery is one of the options in the current treatment guidelines for this chronic, diet-caused disease.
- Maybe it's radical that the majority of Americans continue to eat the S.A.D., even though it is responsible for most of the chronic diseases we suffer and die from (hypertension, high cholesterol, heart attacks and strokes, pre-diabetes and diabetes, inflammatory diseases, autoimmune diseases, dementia, osteoporosis, and many forms of cancer).

DIET, WHAT WE SHOULD BE EATING & DRINKING DAILY

- Maybe it's radical that our nation spent 3.2 trillion dollars on healthcare in 2016, yet we rank far down the list of healthcare outcomes compared to other developed countries. It's estimated that 75 to 80 percent of this cost would be eliminated if we all embraced optimal lifestyle choices.

Now the second issue: Is plant-based nutrition restrictive? Big Food has Americans addicted (literally) to salt, sugar, and fat. So, when people go plant-based, it takes 10 to 14 days for these addictions to resolve, and during that time some people feel deprived. After that though, they lose their taste for the things they shouldn't be eating. Plant-based eating opens up a whole new world of tasty food. Asian, Middle Eastern, East Indian, and many other plant-based cultures have developed delicious dishes, and many American chefs are finally getting on board. There are also many good recipe books, including *Forks Over Knives Cookbook, Oh She Glows, Isa Does It* and *Thug Kitchen*.

From a nutritional point of view, a plant-based diet has all the macronutrients that an animal-based diet does: protein, carbohydrates, and fat. Polyunsaturated fat from plants is a healthy fat compared to saturated and trans fats in animal products, and plant protein has been shown to be healthier for humans than animal protein (search this on *nutritionfacts.org*). A plant-based diet also has fiber, which animal products lack. And only plants have a plethora of health-promoting micronutrients such as antioxidants. When you consider that only 3 percent of Americans get the recommended amount of fiber in their diet, and only a somewhat larger percentage eats the recommended amount of fruit, nuts and vegetables, it is the animal-based diet that seems restrictive.

"We don't have a health care system,
but rather a disease management system
—we wait until diseases occur
and then spend a lot of effort and money
trying to manage them."

– Author unknown

DOPAMINE
AND FOOD CRAVINGS

Regular exercise and a plant-based, whole (unprocessed) food diet with avoidance of salt, sugar, and added oil promotes optimal health and longevity. Why, then, is it so difficult for many people to moderate their lifestyle? One problem is that we are bombarded by advertising from Big Food, and unhealthy food is everywhere. However, the most important factor is the neurotransmitter dopamine, which is produced by the pleasure center in our brain. Joel Fuhrman M.D. says in his new book *Fast Food Genocide* that "overeating and substance/drug abuse share … common characteristics, including tolerance (needing greater amounts over time to reach the same 'high'), unsuccessful efforts to cut back on consumption, and use of the substance despite negative consequences."

In his book *Power Foods for the Brain*, Dr. Neal Barnard points out that there is an evolutionary reason we and other primates have dopamine: "Your reward center is looking for food and for a receptive mate, and when it finds them, out comes the dopamine. But this primitive system can be hijacked by drugs" such as marijuana, cocaine, heroin, and other narcotics. Wine, cigarettes, and coffee all trigger dopamine, as do the following foods, known as "comfort foods:"

• Sugar, which is difficult for many people to give up.
• Chocolate is another.
• Cows' milk (Dr. Barnard says that in your digestive tract, milk's casein protein "breaks apart to release mild opiates, called casomorphins," which trigger dopamine release.)
• Cheese "has concentrated casein and so delivers a much larger casomorphin dose." Unfortunately, cheese is loaded with calories, saturated fat and sodium, "but people flock to the cheese counter to get their hit of opiates and dopamine." No wonder many people adapting a plant-based lifestyle have difficulty giving up cheese.
• Meat triggers dopamine release. When people are given an opiate blocker, they lose interest in meat.
• According to Dr. Fuhrman, refined/junk food, fast food and oils all trigger the dopamine response.

All humans have a gene called DRD2 (dopamine receptor D2), which Dr. Barnard says is "involved in building the receptors for dopamine." People with a variant of this gene have one-third fewer dopamine receptors, and they "need an extra amount of dopamine just to feel normal." Interestingly, in a study conducted by Dr. Barnard, half of diabetic patients had this variant. This contributed to these people overeating unhealthy food, becoming overweight and diabetic.

Food manufacturers take advantage of the dopamine effect. They hire scientists to figure out how to make their food more addictive to people, just like tobacco companies did a few decades ago with cigarettes. Food companies are more concerned with their bottom line than your health, and have Americans addicted to salt, sugar, and fat. Dr. Fuhrman says that fast foods "rich in added sweeteners, salt, oils, and artificial flavoring (called 'highly palatable foods' by food scientists) have addictive properties. Eating a little makes you want more." Restaurant owners also use food addictions to their benefit.

So, what to do? If you adopt a plant-based diet, your food addictions will disappear in 10 to 14 days, and your taste buds will change. Your desire to eat will then be driven by need for calories, rather than food cravings. Another approach is to do what Paul McCartney and his wife did: overcome craving for animal products by developing compassion for animals. As they were eating lamb roast for Sunday brunch one day, they looked at the cute, playful lambs outside the window of their farmhouse and decided to give up meat. Other people make the decision to eat healthier so they can be around to see their grandchildren grow up, or because they know that eating plants instead of meat has much less of an environmental impact. An important part of eating healthier is to exercise, which increases your own "feel good" chemicals—endorphins.

DOPAMINE

"There's one thing we know for sure: raw vegetables and fresh fruits have powerful anti-cancer agents."

– Joel Fuhrman, M.D.

HOW WHAT WE EAT AFFECTS THE PLANET

According to an article in the respected British medical journal *Lancet*, climate change is the biggest global health threat of the 21st century. We physicians need to speak out on this. The August 5, 2018 Sunday *New York Times* devoted the entire magazine section to a comprehensive article on global warming. The title is "Thirty years ago, we could have saved the planet." At one time climate change was a bipartisan issue—since it affects all of us it still should be. The article makes it disturbingly clear that the planet our children and grandchildren will inherit won't be as livable as it is today, and eventually human civilization will be at risk.

Therefore, it's imperative that people become aware of how their food choices affect the environment. There's no question that eating plants, which are at the bottom of the food chain, has much less of an environmental impact than eating animal products. The non-profit Environmental Working Group (EWG) notes that "production, processing and distribution of meat requires huge outlays of pesticide, fertilizer, fuel, feed and water while releasing greenhouse gasses, manure and a range of toxic chemicals into our air and water."

An article in *Scientific American* noted that raising red meat such as beef and lamb are responsible for 10 to 40 times more greenhouse gasses than growing vegetables and grains. Another way to look at this is that it takes 25 kcal of fossil fuel energy to produce 1 kcal of animal protein, whereas it takes 2.2 kcal to produce 1 kcal of protein from grains. Following are the number of kilograms of greenhouse gas resulting from production of 100 grams of various foods: beef: 50; poultry: 5.7; tofu: 2.

An article produced by the University of Oxford in collaboration with the LCA Research Group of Switzerland, and published in *Forbes* notes that meat and dairy provide 18 percent of all calories consumed on the planet but account for 83 percent of the farmland and 60 percent of greenhouse gas emissions. It also points out that if the entire world cut out meat and dairy, global farmland would decrease by 75 percent; the equivalent of the land mass of the U.S., China, European Union, and Australia combined would go from farmland back to its natural state.

Other environmental issues associated with consumption of animal products include:

- A 2009 study indicated that 4/5 of deforestation across the Amazon is linked to cattle ranching.
- Factory farms create huge amounts of sewage waste, which causes water pollution.
- Antibiotics are used in factory and even conventional farming to prevent disease and to make animals grow faster, which contributes to antibiotic resistance.
- As the world gets hotter and more crowded, water is becoming scarcer. Raising a pound of beef takes multiple times more water than raising a pound of kale.
- Cattle are responsible for 20 percent of the world's methane, a particularly potent greenhouse gas

Authors of the *Forbes* article conclude by saying this: "A vegan diet is the single biggest way to reduce your impact on Earth. Buying an electric car, lowering your thermostat, taking quick showers all pale in comparison to simply eating less meat and dairy. Particularly, reducing the consumption of beef, dairy, and pork cuts out some of the largest culprits." We know that a plant-based diet is best for optimal human health; it is also best for the health of our planet. Or as Dr. Greger puts it on *nutritionfacts.org*, "meat is heat."

ENVIRONMENT

"We live in the land of plenty,
but most Americans have nutritional deficiencies
—in fiber, and the health-promoting micronutrients
that fruit, vegetables, whole grains, nuts and seeds offer."

- Greg Feinsinger, M.D.

EXERCISE IS IMPORTANT FOR OPTIMAL HEALTH

Dr. Greger, in his book *How Not to Die,* recommends ideally 90 minutes of moderate exercise or 40 minutes of vigorous activity daily. However, other experts point out that even 30 minutes a day of brisk walking is very beneficial. Examples of moderate exercise are biking on the level, dancing, downhill skiing, hiking, housework, roller-skating, light snow shoveling, recreational swimming, brisk walking (4 mph), yard work, and yoga. Examples of vigorous activities include bicycling uphill, circuit weight-training, cross-country skiing, racquetball, running, singles tennis, swimming laps, and walking briskly uphill. Recent evidence indicates that interval training once or twice a week adds additional benefit, meaning pushing yourself hard enough to get your heart and respiratory rate up for 3 to 4 minutes at a time, repeat 3 times, with a brief rest in between.

Among the many health benefits of exercise are that it:

- Helps overweight people lose weight and other people maintain ideal body weight
- Lowers blood pressure
- Can prevent and reverse type 2 diabetes
- Improves endothelial function (referring to the organ system that lines your arteries)

Some benefits of endothelial health are:

- Decreases the risk of heart attacks and strokes
- Decreases the risk of several types of cancer
- Maintains joint health and range of motion
- Creates strong bones and muscles
- Helps prevent and treat depression
- Helps prevent dementia including Alzheimer's
- Improves low back pain
- Helps people live longer, but more importantly enhances quality of life as they age

Some caveats about exercise are:

- If you think you don't have time to exercise, even 10 minutes of walking 3 times a day is beneficial.
- If you sit for prolonged periods watching TV or at a sedentary job, you undo a lot of the benefit of exercise. So get up and move about at least every 30 minutes, or use a standup desk.
- A lot of aging is loss of strength, which starts at around age 40. So, if you are 40 or over, engage in strength training twice a week.
- If you have chest pain or unusual shortness of breath while exercising, stop immediately and go to the E.R.
- If you have known heart disease, or multiple risk factors, check with your PCP or cardiologist before starting an exercise program.
- Never engage in vigorous exercise within 2 hours after eating, while your heart is pumping blood to your digestive system.
- Especially if you are over 40 it's dangerous to be a "weekend warrior"—couch potato all week and then exercise vigorously on the weekend.
- There is such a thing as too much exercise. Marathoners have evidence of heart damage after running an event, and people who run marathons frequently, or even occasional ultra-marathons or full iron-man triathlons are at higher risk for atrial fibrillation. These over-exercisers are also at higher risk for atherosclerosis, the cause of heart attacks and strokes—at least in part due to the oxidative stress that intense, prolonged exercises causes.
- Taking antioxidant pills does not help with the oxidative stress of "too much exercise," but eating foods high in antioxidants does (fruits and vegetables). Read *Eat and Run* by famous ultra-marathoner Scott Jurek to learn more.

"The modern diet is grossly deficient in hundreds of important plant-derived immunity-building compounds."

– Joel Fuhrman, M.D.

IS THERE SUCH A THING AS TOO MUCH EXERCISE?

The evidence is clear that regular exercise has many health benefits. It decreases the risk of heart attacks, strokes, type 2 diabetes, osteoporosis, and many forms of cancer. It lowers weight and blood pressure, helps with sleep, and relieves stress and depression. People who exercise live longer and have better quality of life as they age.

Most authorities recommend moderate-intensity aerobic exercise such as brisk walking (4 miles per hour) for at least 30 minutes a day, but only a minority of Americans achieve this. Additional benefit occurs with 60 minutes a day and even more with 90 minutes. I tell patients to walk at least 30 minutes a day, fast enough so that they could talk but not sing. People age 40 and over need to also do strength training (e.g. resistance bands, light weights, kettlebell) for 20 minutes twice a week, on non-consecutive days. The reason for this is that loss of strength starts at around 40, which contributes to aging. If you exercise but sit at a desk the rest of the day, that undoes the benefit of exercise, so use a standup desk and/or walk around every 30 minutes.

Beyond about 90 minutes a day of moderate exercise, or lesser amounts of intense exercise, the risks may outweigh the benefits. How to define too much exercise varies with the exerciser, but as a Supreme Court justice once said about pornography, "you know it when you see it." An excellent book on this subject is *The Haywire Heart, How Too Much Exercise Can Kill You, And What You Can Do To Protect Your Heart*. The authors are John Mandrola, M.D. a cardiac electrophysiologist (a cardiologist who sub-specializes in problems of the electrical conduction system of the heart); Chris Case, editor of VeloNews; and Lennard Zinn who custom-makes bicycles in Boulder, Colorado. All three are elite athletes, and Lennard Zinn has a personal history of a heart arrhythmia, which he attributes to over-exercise.

The most common cause of death in the U.S. is heart attacks, caused by rupture of atherosclerotic plaque in a coronary (heart) artery. There's evidence that in general heavy exercisers develop more plaque than non-exercisers, but their plaque tends to be calcified and more stable. So far there is no evidence that these athletes are at increased risk for heart attacks (non-athletic people with high calcium scores are).

Prolonged/intense exercise has been shown to cause elevation of cardiac enzymes such as troponin, indicating damage to cardiac muscle. This kind of exercise can also result in small scars that can interfere with the heart's electrical conduction system. Over-exercisers are more prone to rhythm disturbances involving the atria (the two smaller chambers of the heart), such as atrial fibrillation. Scarring can also cause rhythm disturbances in the ventricles (the two larger heart chambers), which can be more dangerous.

So, if you want a long, good-quality life, by all means exercise. If you love intense exercise, and you have a family history of heart disease or sudden death (usually caused by an arrhythmia), you should see a cardiologist before engaging in heavy exercise, even if you are school-aged (the usual pre-participation sports physicals usually don't pick up the congenital problems that cause young athletes to die on the field). If you are 40 or over and intense and/or prolonged exercise has become an important part of your life, realize that as you age you may be taking some risk. At the very least, understand that the older you get the more important rest/recovery days become.

If you are exercising and have chest pain, unusual fatigue or shortness of breath, notice heart speedups out of proportion to the exercise you're doing, feel dizzy or faint, or notice palpitations or an irregular pulse, stop immediately and go to the nearest ER. If the symptoms don't include chest pain and aren't severe, don't exercise again until you see your PCP, a cardiologist, or an electrophysiologist, depending on the circumstances. To learn more, read *The Haywire Heart*.

"The only way you're going to hurt yourself with fruit is if you drop a 20-pound watermelon on your foot."

– Michael Greger, M.D.

MEDICINAL USES OF GINGER

Various plants have been used in different cultures as "folk remedies" for centuries. However, that doesn't necessarily mean they are effective or free of side effects. Scientific studies have been a long time in coming, because they cost money, and Big Pharma, that underwrites studies of pharmaceuticals, can't make money selling plants. Fortunately, in recent years some good, placebo-controlled studies have been done on a number of natural products used in traditional medicine. As expected, some of these remedies have been shown to be effective and others not, and some have been found to have side effects.

Ginger has been used in folk medicine and has recently undergone scientific studies that showed it to be effective for several conditions, and to be free of significant side effects. We know that intensely colored fruits and vegetables have special antioxidant and anti-inflammatory properties, so we tell people to "eat the rainbow." Intensely flavored plants such as herbs and spices share these properties. Ginger is an intensely flavored spice, and is available in root and powdered form in most grocery stores. Based on Dr. Michael Greger's book *How Not to Die,* and his website *nutritionfacts.org,* credible studies show that ginger can do the following:

- Reduce menstrual cramps, which 90 percent of young women complain of, resulting in an estimated 2 billion dollars of lost productivity annually in the U.S. Most women rely on anti-inflammatories such as ibuprofen, but these can have side effects such as stomach irritation and bleeding, hypertension, and increased risk of heart attacks. One-fourth teaspoon of powdered ginger taken 3 times a day works as well as 400 mg. of ibuprofen 3 times a day, with minimal cost and no side-effects.
- Reduce heavy menstrual flow, which many young women complain of. Anti-inflammatories are often used to treat this condition, but 1/8 tsp. of ginger daily for 3 days starting one day before menstrual onset has been shown to cut menstrual flow in half.
- Treat morning sickness, experienced by 70 to 85 percent of pregnant American women. This condition can sometimes be so serious that hospitalization and IV fluids are required. One gram of ginger a day is often effective in treat-

ing morning sickness. This is equivalent to 1/2 teaspoon of powdered ginger, 1 tsp. of grated fresh ginger, or 4 cups of ginger tea. Ginger is safe during pregnancy, although the maximum recommended dose is 4 grams a day. (Note that marijuana is also effective but there are concerns about fetal safety.)

- Treat nausea caused by other conditions. Ginger has been shown to be effective in treating postoperative nausea and vomiting, motion sickness, and nausea associated with HIV anti-retroviral treatment. Ginger has also been shown to prevent nausea associated with chemotherapy.
- Treat migraine headaches. Imitrex (sumatriptan) and similar drugs have become the mainstay of migraine treatment, but are costly and often have side effects, including dizziness, sedation, and heartburn; and have rarely been associated with heart attacks and fatal heart irregularities. One-eighth of a teaspoon of ginger has been shown to be as effective as Imitrex, without the side effects or cost.
- Mitigate radiation damage. Cooked ginger has been shown in the lab and in people to help prevent radiation damage.

"Heart disease is a foodborne illness."

– Caldwell Esselstyn, M.D.

PEPPERMINT FOR IBS
(IRRITABLE BOWEL SYNDROME)
AND MORE

IBS (irritable bowel syndrome), which affects 1 out of 7 Americans, is a chronic, episodic condition characterized by low abdominal cramping, and often either diarrhea or constipation. No one dies from IBS, but it definitely adversely affects quality of life. Diagnosis is based on symptoms; there is no test for IBS, but more serious diseases need to be ruled out when patients present with IBS symptoms.

Pharmaceuticals have never been very successful for treating IBS. Anti-spasmodic drugs and antidepressants were used in the past, but weren't very effective, and had a high rate of side effects. The newer medications can cost up to $3,000 a year, have side effects, and their effectiveness isn't impressive.

Peppermint has been used for thousands of years to treat GI symptoms. After dinner mints not only act as a breath freshener, but also relieve flatus and abdominal cramping associated with the gastro-colic reflex—when the stomach is full, the colon contracts to allow room in the stomach for more food. Peppermint tea does the same thing. In at least one study, peppermint oil capsules were as effective in treating symptoms of IBS, and had no side effects. According to Dr. Greger (*nutritionfacts.org*), 1/4 cup of fresh mint leaves contains the same amount of peppermint oil as the capsules in this study, and he maintains that peppermint should be the first line of treatment for IBS.

Because peppermint relaxes the colon, taking it prior to colonoscopy makes the procedure easier and safer. Perforation of the colon is a rare but serious complication of colonoscopy, and it is less apt to occur if the colon is relaxed.

Following are some other medicinal effects of peppermint:

- It can improve athletic performance, thought to be due to opening up the airways.
- It can relieve nausea. Just the smell of essential oil of spearmint can do this, although it's unclear whether it's the smell of peppermint, the smell of alcohol which is part of the essential oil, or whether it's just taking deep breaths.
- Peppermint has an anti-testosterone effect when taken in large doses, which can lower libido in men—so men should beware. This effect can be useful in

GI, GYN ISSUES

treating women with unwanted hair and with PCOS (polycystic ovarian syndrome), both of which are associated with higher-than-normal testosterone levels.

Although intuitively you'd think that peppermint would work for colic, it should not be given to infants or young children because of potential serious side effects (just because something is natural doesn't necessarily mean it's safe).

"The answer to the American health crisis
is the food that each of us chooses to put in our mouths each day.
It's as simple as that."

– T. Colin Campbell, PhD

GI, GYN ISSUES

CHERRIES FOR GOUT

Gout is a painful, acute arthritis, more common in men than women, that classically affects the joint at the base of the big toe, although it sometimes affects other joints. If gout recurs over several years, it can result in chronic degenerative arthritis. The prevalence of gout in the United States is 3.9 percent, which translates to 8.2 million people.

Gout occurs when uric acid, something we all have in our blood, crystalizes in joints, followed by redness, swelling, and acute pain. There can be a hereditary component, and gout is usually but not always associated with high uric acid levels. Some people have high uric acid levels but never get gout, so exactly why an attack of gout occurs when it does is not completely understood. There are certain drugs that can bring on gout though, such as niacin, diuretics, and aspirin.

For an acute attack of gout, anti-inflammatories such as indomethacin, ibuprofen, or naproxen are often used. For people who can't take these drugs (they can cause stomach bleeding and hypertension), cortisone or colchicine are often used. For people who just have 1 or 2 attacks of gout a year, it makes sense just to treat the attacks as they occur. However, if attacks occur more often, or if they occur in joints other than the big toe, it is wise to do something to prevent future attacks. Typically, allopurinol, which lowers uric acid levels, is used for this. Allopurinol should not be started during an acute attack, and often a low dose of daily colchicine is given with it during the first month, since allopurinol can actually bring on an attack during the first month a person is on it. The other problem with this drug is that it can have rare but serious side effects.

Michael Greger, M.D., on his website *nutritionfacts.org*, cites studies showing that cherries lower uric acid and work just as well as drugs, for treatment of acute attacks of gout, and to prevent attacks. Sweet, red cherries work better than tart or yellow cherries, and the dose is 15 cherries a day. When cherries are not in season, frozen cherries work as well, as does a tablespoonful of cherry juice concentrate twice a day.

Uric acid is a breakdown product of purines, and people with recurrent gout should avoid purine-containing food, such as seafood and meat (particularly sardines and organ meat). People with recurrent gout should also avoid alcohol, particularly beer. A few vegetables also have purines, such as mushrooms and asparagus, but Dr. Greger says that for whatever reason, vegetable sources of purines don't seem to bring on gout attacks, and gout is rare in people who are on a total plant-based diet.

"The most important thing to remember about food labels
is that you should avoid foods that have labels."

– Joel Fuhrman, M.D.

GOUT

WHY AREN'T HEALTH CARE PROVIDERS EDUCATING THEIR PATIENTS ABOUT THE HEALTH BENEFITS OF PLANT-BASED NUTRITION?

What if there were a pill that prevented and reversed heart disease, hypertension, high cholesterol, and type 2 diabetes; prevented up to 60 percent of cancer; prevented kidney stones and osteoporosis and gout; reduced the incidence of inflammatory diseases such as rheumatoid arthritis; reduced dementia, including Alzheimer's; and reduced the incidence of autoimmune diseases such as type 1 diabetes and M.S.? And what if it had no side effects and cost no more than what people already spend on groceries every day? Health care providers would all know about this drug due to marketing by the company that made it, and the public would be aware of it and demand it. Obviously health care providers would prescribe it and would be accused of malpractice if they didn't.

Well there is such a treatment but it isn't a pill. Rather it's lifestyle modification consisting of a plant-based, whole (unprocessed) foods, low-fat (PBWFLF) diet, plus regular exercise. Unfortunately, most people don't know about this option and their health care providers don't educate them about it. According to Dr. Greger (*nutritionfacts.org*), here are some of the reasons why:

- Performing surgical interventions such as stents and bypass have the potential for enormous financial reward for hospitals and for the providers who do them.
- Doctors don't get training in nutrition in medical school and most don't know much if anything about it. There was a study comparing doctors' knowledge to patients' knowledge of nutrition, and the patients won.
- Even if a doctor does know something about nutrition, he or she doesn't get paid much for counseling and is often rushed and doesn't have the time to do it.
- Doctors assume that patients won't adopt lifestyle modification, but that is the old, paternalistic way of practicing medicine. Our job should be to present the various options to the patient and let them decide what they want to do.
- Medical studies, medical schools, medical journals, and medical conferences often get funding from the pharmaceutical and the food industries.

- Committees that make up national guidelines on nutrition and medical practices (e.g. hypertension, cholesterol, diabetes guidelines for physicians) usually have members who represent the pharmaceutical and food industry.
- These days, physicians who give presentations at medical conferences have to disclose what ties they have to pharmaceutical and other companies and it's amazing how long the list often is.
- Doctors often have a "slavish devotion" to orthodoxy. The average time it takes for medical practice to change from the time the science tells us we should change is 17 years!

It is true that in the setting of a heart attack, a stent can save your life. But other than that situation, stents and bypass surgery have not been shown to save lives or improve quality of life when compared to lifestyle modification. Stents are invasive and occasionally can result in serious complications. Bypass surgery is much more invasive and can result in complications including permanent brain damage and death. Furthermore, these procedures cost the medical system billions of dollars a year. And 100,000 people die in America every year from adverse reactions to drugs.

Furthermore, eating a plant-based diet is better for the planet. To produce 1 pound of beef it takes 1,847 gallons of water; to produce 1 pound of broccoli takes 34 gallons. The carbon dioxide footprint to produce 1 pound of beef is 39.2, whereas for lentils it is 0.9. And then there is the issue of inhumane treatment of animals in factory farming.

So clearly, all doctors should feel obligated to learn about nutrition and to discuss lifestyle intervention as an option for their patients. This is the right thing for them to do for their patients, to help do something about our unsustainable and expensive medical system, and for the planet. Sure, not all patients are going to be willing to go totally plant-based, but in my experience many will, and the rest will at least make some changes. There is some hope. A recent president of the American College of Cardiology became vegan after looking at the facts and determining this was the healthiest way to go. And a colleague of mine recently attended a conference for plant-based cardiologists!

HEALTH CARE SYSTEM—PROBLEMS WITH

THE THIRD CAUSE OF DEATH IN THE U.S.

Most people who go into medicine do so because they want to help others. And all doctors are aware of the part of the Hippocratic oath that says first do no harm. However, the medical field has a dirty little secret: More than 250,000 deaths a year in the U.S. are caused by mistakes by the American health care system, making this the third leading cause of death, after number one–heart disease and number two–cancer.

In his book *How Not to Die,* Dr. Greger devotes a chapter to how not to die from iatrogenic causes, iatrogenic referring to doctor-caused. Here are the pertinent facts:

- Side effects from medications given in hospitals kill approximately 106,000 Americans every year, and another 199,000 deaths occur from outpatient prescription drugs (this figure does not include deaths from prescription narcotics or intentional overdoses).
- At least 7,000 people die in hospitals every year from being given the wrong medication by mistake.
- Some 20,000 patients die annually from other hospital errors.
- Hospital-acquired infections result in 99,000 deaths a year. Given this, it's unconscionable that care workers are only 50 percent compliant with hand-washing recommendations, with studies showing that doctors are the worst offenders.
- Twelve thousand patients die every year of complications from operations that were unnecessary in the first place, let alone patients who die from complications from operations deemed "necessary."
- Radiation from studies such as CT scans and nuclear cardiac stress tests is estimated to cause thousands of cancer deaths every year. Often these studies are unnecessary and patients aren't informed about the risks of radiation or about safer alternatives.
- Diagnostic errors contribute to 10 percent of iatrogenic patient deaths.
- Forty-five percent of patients don't receive the recommended treatment for their condition. For example, many studies show that when patients are discharged from hospitals after heart attacks, a large percentage don't receive all the guideline-recommended treatments, whether their caregivers are cardiologists or primary care doctors.

HEALTH CARE SYSTEM—PROBLEMS WITH

• Often when primary care physicians see patients for follow-up visits after discharge from the hospital, they don't have the documents such as discharge summaries needed for appropriate continuity of care. A 2009 study showed that 30 percent of hospitalized Medicare patients were readmitted within 30 days.

An eye-opening, well-written book worth reading is *How Doctors Think,* by Jerome Groopman, a hematologist and oncologist. One of the stories in it is about a patient named Anne, who at age 20 started having severe abdominal cramps, nausea, and diarrhea whenever she ate. This led to significant weight loss and malnutrition including an impaired immune system, and she came close to dying. She saw multiple doctors over the years, including specialists, and underwent a multitude of tests. Eventually she was diagnosed with anorexia and bulimia and was sent to psychiatrists. After years of this, she finally saw a specialist who sat down with her and took the time to listen to her complete story (good medicine is not always about expensive tests) and diagnosed her celiac sprue, which was confirmed by appropriate tests. He told her to go on a gluten-free diet and soon she was well and has remained so. Personally, I have had one negative encounter with the medical system: When I was a freshman at Oberlin College I developed low abdominal pain. I went to the college physician (students called him "Max the Axe") who examined me and told me I was constipated and to go back to my dorm room and take an enema, which I did. The next day I felt worse and late in the afternoon went back to the student health clinic. I told the nurse I was worse but she told me the clinic was closing for the day and to come back the next morning. Luckily, I had the presence of mind to see a private surgeon in town that evening and within an hour I was on the operating table with a ruptured appendix, a condition that people still die from to this day.

We all have had or know people who have had experiences like this. Having discussions like this is not doctor-bashing (I am proud to be a physician and feel fortunate to be in a field where I can help people). However, we doctors could, should, and must take ownership of these problems and make the necessary changes so that medical mistakes are maybe the one hundredth cause of death instead of the third. Obamacare includes incentives to avoid medical errors. A few hospitals in the country have taken aggressive steps in this direction, with good results. And all hospitals have taken at least some steps to correct iatrogenic deaths, such as encouraging hand washing and developing systems to prevent surgeons from operating on the wrong extremity. Some medical system analysts think that medicine should be run more like the airlines, with checklists. This shouldn't be that hard to institute, with modern technology such as computers. But in medicine, there is always a lot of inertia due to a desire to maintain the status quo, even if the status quo involves tens of thousands of patient deaths.

One option of course is to limit our contact with the medical system by taking better care of ourselves, with daily exercise and optimal diet.

HOW TO MINIMIZE ERRORS WHEN ENGAGING WITH THE AMERICAN HEALTH CARE SYSTEM

The September 2017 issue of the *AARP Bulletin* had an article with the title "12 Ways The Health Care System May Be Harming You," which included ways patients can be proactive in preventing medical mistakes. Dr. Michael Greger's book *How Not to Die* has a chapter about how not to die from iatrogenic (doctor-caused) harm. *How Doctors Think* is a thoughtful, eye-opening book written by oncologist Jerome Groopman, M.D., about why doctors make diagnostic errors. Based on these sources and my 42 years of family practice, here are some tips for patients to help prevent medical errors:

- Be sure your doctor is compassionate, thorough, up-to-date, and competent. The latter two qualities are more likely if he or she is board-certified.
- The most important factor in making a correct diagnosis is the history the patient gives. Your doctor will want to know what your symptoms are, when they began, if anything makes them worse such as eating or exercise. Present your story in a concise manner, and use notes if you need to so you don't forget important facts. To allow your doctor to focus on your primary issue, don't take up office visit time with unhelpful, extraneous data.
- A thorough doctor will want to know about your past medical history, family history of pertinent medical problems, and a social history (e.g. history of smoking, alcohol use, exercise, and eating habits). So if your mother died from colon cancer at age 50, your doctor needs to know that, but taking up office visit time talking about a cousin who died in an MVA won't be helpful.
- I always had patients bring their prescription meds, over-the-counter meds, and any supplements they were taking to office visits. Often patients weren't taking exactly what I or they thought they were taking.
- Have a clear understanding about your doctor's diagnosis. Go home and look it up on the Internet and be sure the diagnosis jives with your symptoms and that the plan of treatment seems reasonable.
- If you aren't getting better, make an appointment for a recheck and ask your

doctor if it is possible you have something else. Ask for a second opinion if you are left with unanswered questions or concerns.

- Keep in mind that tests are not always accurate. For example, you can have a normal fasting blood sugar and still have diabetes. Even X-ray and biopsy reports can be inaccurate (for example the biopsy needle can miss the cancer).
- If tests that involve radiation are recommended, such as CT scans or nuclear imaging, ask if there are radiation-free alternatives (e.g. MRI instead of a CT scan). Radiation is cumulative and is harmful and especially if you are seeing more than one doctor, nobody but you is keeping track of how much radiation you are being exposed to over the years.
- Health care providers including doctors fail to wash their hands when they should 50 percent of the time, which contributes to the 99,000 deaths that occur every year from hospital-acquired infections. So especially if you're in the hospital, if a provider is about to examine you without washing their hands, request that they do so.
- Seven thousand people die annually in hospitals from being given the wrong medication. If you're hospitalized, be sure that the nurse checks your identification bracelet before giving you anything by mouth, by injection, or IV.
- Side effects from medications given in the hospital result in 106,000 deaths annually, so before being given anything ask what it's for and understand the necessity.
- Outpatient prescription drug side effects result in some 199,000 deaths every year. So if your doctor recommends medication, ask if there are alternatives such as lifestyle modification (e.g. exercise and plant-based nutrition can reverse type 2 diabetes). A large percentage of antibiotic prescriptions that are written are not appropriate.
- If a doctor recommends surgery and the situation is not an emergency, consider a second opinion. Surgery is never the perfect answer, because complications such as post-op infections and even death can occur. If you have acute appendicitis or a perforated bowel, there is no question that surgery can save your life. But many hysterectomies, many back surgeries, small hernia repairs, and repairing degenerative meniscus tears in the elderly are examples of operations that are much more questionable.

Modern medicine offers us cures that we never dreamed of years ago, and we are lucky it is available when we need it. But the history of medicine has a dark side in that many standards of care in the past were later found to be harmful and unnecessary. For example, decades ago, enlarged tonsils were sometimes treated with radiation, which was later found to cause cancer of the head and neck. Doctors used to remove the whole meniscus when a small tear occurred, which caused knee arthritis. Radical mastectomies, a very disfiguring operation, were done for years for breast cancer, and were later found to be unnecessary. Currently, cardiac stents and coronary bypass surgery are done frequently, even though they have never been shown to save lives (the exception being a stent in the setting of an acute heart attack) or improve quality of life when compared to aggressive medical therapy and/or lifestyle modification. And bypass surgery in particular can result in serious complications, including death.

The best thing you can do to avoid doctor and hospital-caused deaths is to avoid need for medical care by staying healthy: by exercising regularly and eating an optimal diet. Seventy-five to 80 percent of the chronic diseases we suffer from in Western societies are preventable by lifestyle modification, and if you already have one or more of them, most are reversible. We're talking here about obesity, hypertension, high cholesterol, diabetes, cardiovascular disease, dementia, autoimmune diseases, inflammatory diseases, osteoporosis, and even many forms of cancer. These account for the large majority of doctor and hospital visits and of the 3.2 trillion dollars (!) spent in 2016 on health care in this country.

"Medicines cannot drug away
the cellular defects that develop in response
to improper nutrition throughout life."

– Joel Fuhrman, M.D.

MEDICAL DEVICES ARE POORLY REGULATED, CAN CAUSE HARM

Medical devices range from robots that perform surgery to lens implants, cardiac stents and pacemakers. The medical device industry is a 300-billion-dollar-a-year industry, that has even more influence in Washington than Big Pharm—in 2017 they spent 64 million on lobbying. I attended a showing at Paepcke Auditorium in Aspen of a documentary available on Netflix called *The Bleeding Edge*. The director, Kirby Dick, was there for an interview and Q and A after the showing. The film is about the poor regulation of the medical device industry, and how this is causing harm to patients.

Most people, including doctors who recommend or use medical devices, assume that the FDA uses the same scrutiny for these devices that it does for pharmaceuticals. However, that's not the case; many new devices that come on the market haven't been proven to be effective or safe in humans. Following are 4 examples from *The Bleeding Edge* that illustrate the problem.

Essure is a small metal coil used for female sterilization. The coil is placed in women's fallopian tubes in an office setting, and it induces scarring, which prevents sperm from entering the tubes. The device was developed by Conceptus, which was later bought by Bayer. It was approved by the FDA in 2002, based on short-term studies of fewer than 1 or 2 years, even though it was intended for lifetime use. In the last several years, thousands of women have complained of side effects, including perforations of their tubes; chronic pain; and bleeding (sometimes leading to hysterectomies); plus hundreds of unintended pregnancies. One of the problems with this device is that in some women it causes an autoimmune response, which results in several other symptoms including headaches and feeling crummy. Many Essure devices have had to be removed, although removal is difficult (you can't just pull them out when scar tissue has formed). Bayer finally announced it would halt U.S. sales by the end of the year. In the meantime, Bayer is paying out millions of dollars for lawsuits, but is still making billions of dollars by continuing to sell the product.

There are several types of hip replacements, including metal-on-metal cobalt devices. An orthopedist in Alaska was featured in *The Bleeding Edge*, who had this type of replacement himself, and later developed multiple symptoms, including brain fog,

148

and eventually a complete mental breakdown. His blood level of cobalt was 100 times the normal limit. The joint replacement was removed—with difficulty—and replaced with another type of device. Within a month his symptoms resolved. There are 10 million people worldwide with cobalt hip, knee, and shoulder replacements, and it turns out that many of these people are suffering from similar symptoms. Problems have also occurred with cobalt-on-polyethylene implants. If you have a cobalt-containing implant, have your blood cobalt level checked periodically.

Polypropylene mesh has been used for years for hernia repairs, and in recent years it has been marketed under the brand name Prolift by Ethicon, a subsidiary of Johnson and Johnson, for pelvic floor laxity in middle-aged and older women— often related to the trauma of childbirth. It costs $25 to make, but is sold for $2,000. It was introduced in 2005, bypassing FDA scrutiny due to being similar to the previously-approved hernia mesh. Prolift causes an inflammatory response and scarring, and as the scar matures, the tissues with which it comes in contact contract, creating a "rigid, hard object" around the vagina, bladder and urethra (the tube urine passes though as it exits the bladder). Many women who underwent this procedure started complaining of pain and other symptoms. Their complaints were brushed off by doctors, but eventually complaints became severe and numerous enough that they could no longer be ignored. Unfortunately, it's essentially impossible to remove all the mesh in a patient with complaints, due to scar tissue in and around it. According to the documentary, the surgeons who developed prototypes knew there were problems, but marketing was already underway, and "marketing won out over science." Currently, Johnson and Johnson has been hit with 300 million dollars in lawsuits, but keeps marketing their product because of 683 billion in profits.

The Da Vinci is a robotic surgical system that costs 2 million dollars, made by Intuitive Surgical. It was cleared by the FDA in 2000, and is used for operations such as prostatectomies and hysterectomies. There is a long learning curve for surgeons wanting to become adept at using this technology, and when the Da Vinci first came out, 2 weeks of intense training was promised for each surgeon who was going to use it. Within a short time, the training was reduced to 2 days, and the company's reps pushed surgeons into using the technology before they were proficient. One surgeon in the film, who is an expert in robotic surgery, stated that it took him 200–300 procedure before he felt proficient. Serious complications have occurred using the Da Vinci System, including vaginal cuff dehiscence in gyn procedures, where closure of the incision at the top of the vagina following a hysterectomy fails, in some instances resulting in women's intestines falling into and protruding from their vaginas. Of note is that robotic surgery is more expensive, takes longer, and has poorer results than traditional surgery.

The film makes the following suggestions for protecting yourself before someone puts a medical device in you or when a surgeon suggests robotic surgery: (1) Do your own research on the device. (2) Get a second opinion. (3) Find out how many procedures the surgeon has done. (4) Have a patient advocate come with you to your appointments. (5) Go to *openpaymentdata.cms.gov* to see if the surgeon has a financial interest in the recommended medical device. (6) Keep in mind that new, cutting edge technology isn't necessarily better. (7) Realize that surgeons often have cozy relationships with medical device reps, who influence their recommendations.

Medical devices such as pacemakers for serious cardiac rhythm disturbances, and stents for a heart attack, can save your life. But some medical devices can make you sick and even kill you. These devices all need to be proven to be effective and safe before they are used in humans, and physicians using them need to be properly trained.

*"People who are lonely and depressed
are three to ten times more likely to get sick and die prematurely
than those who have a strong sense of love and community."*

– Dean Ornish, M.D.

WE NEED TO FIX OUR EXPENSIVE, BROKEN HEALTH CARE SYSTEM

A better term than health care system would be disease management system; we wait until diseases occur and then we spend a lot of effort and money trying to manage them (3.2 trillion dollars in 2016). Not only is our health care system expensive, it's also deadly; complications and errors in our health care system are the third cause of death in America, following heart attacks and cancer.

The PNHP (Physicians for a National Health Plan) organization notes that:

- "The USA spends twice as much per person on healthcare as other industrialized nations, yet we rank near the bottom in nearly all health indicators (including life expectancy and infant and maternal mortality)."
- "Each year, one trillion of our healthcare dollars go to administrative costs (31 percent)." Although counterintuitive for some people, the administrative costs for government programs such as Medicare are only a fraction of the costs for private programs.
- "Our prescription drug prices are the highest in the world. Congress prohibited Medicare from negotiating drug prices." (Due to the power Big Pharma has in Washington.)
- "Thirty million Americans still have no health insurance and another 40 million are underinsured."
- "Most U.S. household bankruptcies are due mainly to medical bills—and most of those households had health insurance."

The book *An American Sickness, How Healthcare Became Big Business and How You Can Take It Back* was written by Elisabeth Rosenthal, M.D., a physician and journalist. She talks about "the transformation of American medicine in a little over a quarter century from a caring endeavor to the most profitable industry in the United States—what many experts refer to as a medical-industrial complex." Following are Dr. Rosenthal's "economic rules of the dysfunctional medical market."

- "More treatment is always better. Default to the most expensive option."
- "A lifetime of treatment is preferable to a cure."

- "Amenities and marketing matter more than good care."
- "As technologies age, prices can rise rather than fall."
- "There is no free choice. Patients are stuck. And they're stuck buying American."
- "More competitors vying for business doesn't mean better prices; it can drive prices up, not down."
- "Economies of scale don't translate to lower prices. With their market power, big providers can simply demand more."
- "There is no such thing as a fixed price for a procedure or test. And the uninsured pay the highest prices of all."
- "There are no standards for billing. There's money to be made in billing for anything and everything."
- "Prices will rise to whatever the market will bear."

Why do we Americans struggle to do what so many other developed countries have done: develop a medical system that covers all our citizens, that is reasonably priced, and that has better outcomes? The answer is at least in part what Dr. Robert Pearl calls the legacy players, in his book *Mistreated, Why We Think We're Getting Good Health Care—and Why We're Usually Wrong*. The legacy players are hospitals, medical insurance companies, the pharmaceutical and medical device industry, and specialty medical societies—all of which resist change because they are deriving huge profits from the current, broken system.

> "Food is really and truly
> the most effective medicine."
>
> – Joel Fuhrman, M.D.

STAND UP FOR YOUR FINANCIAL RIGHTS WHEN DEALING WITH THE AMERICAN HEALTH CARE SYSTEM

In the early 1970s, the American Hospital Association developed a Patient Bill of Rights. This included rights such as "understandable information concerning diagnosis, treatment and prognosis" and a "smoke-free environment."

We now live in an era of exorbitant medical costs, with too many people who don't have insurance coverage or have high deductibles. Therefore, patients need a financial bill of rights. Elisabeth Rosenthal, M.D., is a physician-journalist who wrote a book called *American Sickness, How Healthcare Became Big Business and How You Can Take It Back*. She wrote an opinion piece in the April 27, 2018 Sunday Review section of the *New York Times*, with the title "Nine rights every patient should demand." She recommends that patients are entitled to the following:

- "The right to an itemized bill in plain English" so that patients can "detect and refute improper charges." Medical bills are often not itemized, often include language and abbreviations that lay people can't decipher, and studies show that 30 to 50 percent of medical bills contain errors.
- "The right to never receive a surprise out-of-network bill." This refers to, for example, the hospital being in network but the anesthesia or radiologist isn't, and the patient is unaware of this until they get the bill.
- "The right to accurate information about the provider in-network insurance plans." This addresses the problem of some doctors being in network for certain procedures but not for others (e.g. gastroenterologist in network for polyp removal but not for screening colonoscopy).
- "The right to a stable network." If a doctor or insurer stops participating in a network within the year after an insurance policy is purchased, the patient should still be billed as an in-network patient.
- "The right to be informed of conflicts of interest." Some doctors have a financial stake in testing facilities (e.g. orthopedists owning their own MRI) or procedure facilities such as outpatient surgical centers, which can lead to unnecessary tests and procedures.

- "The right to be informed in advance about any facility fees." For example, if a procedure is done in a doctor's office there is usually no facility fee, but if it is done in the hospital there is. Cost differences associated with different options are seldom discussed with patients.
- "The right to see a price list for elective procedures." Informed consent "should include financial liability as well as medical risk."
- "The right to be informed of cheaper options." For example, months of hospital-based PT are usually ordered following hip replacements, but patients should be told that another, much cheaper option is to have a few instructional sessions and then do the exercises at a gym.
- "The right to know that a disputed bill will not be sent to a collection agency." Dr. Rosenthal points out that hospitals often threaten patients in a way that would be considered extortion in any other business.

Years ago, medicine was a paternalistic profession, and patients did whatever the doctor told them to do, without asking questions. Currently, the practice of medicine is more of a partnership between doctor and patient, with various diagnostic and treatment options being discussed with the patient and a joint decision made before proceeding. Unfortunately, finances are often left out of doctor-patient discussions and this contributes to the high cost of our health care system and to financial hardships for patients. So, ask questions such as whether you really need that MRI or other expensive tests, and about less expensive treatment options such as having a minor procedure done in the doctor's office rather than a hospital. Stand up for your financial rights. Hospitals charge a lot because they can get away with it.

"The human body has no more need for cows' milk
than it does for dogs' milk, horses' milk, or giraffes' milk."

— Dr. Michael Klaper

WHAT YOU AND YOUR PHYSICIAN CAN DO TO COMBAT HIGH PHARMACEUTICAL PRICES

People with insurance often aren't aware of the cost of pharmaceuticals, but high drug costs contribute to high insurance premiums. Physicians often are not aware of the cost of drugs they prescribe. Unfortunately, Big Pharma has powerful lobbyists in Washington and makes large campaign contributions to legislators, so the system is tilted in their favor.

The July 2017 issue of the *American Family Physician* had an editorial about "Drug Price Gouging: When Will It End?" They listed the following suggestions for health care professionals:

- Always prescribe generics when available.
- Learn the cost of non-generic medications you prescribe, when no generics are available.
- Stop justifying prescribing high-cost drugs by assuming that insurance will pay for them so it doesn't matter. It does matter, because expensive drugs increase the cost of medical care for all of us.
- Shun samples left by pharmaceutical reps, because they are brand-name and usually expensive. There is a good argument that drug reps shouldn't be allowed in physician offices.
- Refer patients to assistance programs: RxAssist (*http://rxassist.org/*) and NeedyMeds (*http://rxassist.org*).
- Do not use new drugs until they have been out for a while and have proven to be safe and cost-effective.

Here are my suggestions for what patients can do:

- The best way to beat Big Pharma at their own game is to exercise regularly and eat an optimal diet, therefore eliminating, or at least reducing the need for medications.
- Always request generics from your provider.
- Have your doctor prescribe a higher dose and cut pills in half with a pill split-

ter. Pharmaceutical companies caution against doing this but that advice is given so they can sell more pills.

- If your medications aren't covered by insurance, buy your drugs from Canada. This is illegal in the U.S., thanks to lobbying by Big Pharma, but the Obama administration turned a blind eye, and people do this all the time. To be sure you're dealing with a reputable pharmacy, go to *www.AccessCanadianPharmacy.com.*
- Lobby Washington to do away with laws that prevent Medicare from negotiating for the best drug prices.
- Lobby Washington to prevent new "me too" drugs, which add cost to the system without benefit to patients.
- Lobby Washington to prevent direct marketing of drugs to patients (TV and magazine ads).
- Lobby Washington to institute universal, single-payer health care ("Medicare for all") with medication coverage (yes, some of us will pay higher taxes but it's the right thing to do and we'll all benefit).

The American Family Physician editorial mentions a potential problem that would adversely affect all of us: As part of the current administration's goal of eliminating regulations, they "plan to have the FDA approve drugs that seem safe but whose effectiveness has not been proven. This would take us back to the days of snake oil, only at greatly increased expense, when products could be promoted without proof they worked."

"Moderation kills."

– Caldwell Esselstyn, M.D.

(Moderation is important for certain aspects of life but not for nutrition—people on the Mediterranean diet, a "moderate" diet, still die from heart attacks, whereas people on a plant-based, whole food diet with no salt, sugar or added oil don't.)

SIGNS THAT THE MEDICAL ESTABLISHMENT MAY BE STARTING TO GET HEALTHY EATING

In the 1940s Dr. Walter Kempner proved that severe hypertension could be reversed by diet. Over 25 years ago, Dr. Dean Ornish, and later Dr. Caldwell Esselstyn, proved that our biggest killer—heart disease—can be reversed by plant-based, whole food nutrition with avoidance of salt, sugar, and added oil. But unfortunately, the medical field is bound by tradition; doctors are paid well to do procedures but not for counseling; and physician training and practice are unduly influenced by the pharmaceutical and food industries. As a result, the power of food to prevent and reverse disease has been neglected by traditional medicine.

Finally, there are some hopeful signs that this may be changing. Dr. Kim Williams, who was recently the president of the American Collage of Cardiology, decided to go plant-based a few years ago, after reviewing several different diets. When people asked him why, he said "I don't mind dying so much, but I don't want it to be my fault."

The American Heart Association publishes the respected medical journal *Circulation*. In the June 5, 2018 issue there was an article titled "Medical Nutrition Education, Training and Competencies to Advance Guideline-Based Diet Counseling by Physicians." The article notes that "training physicians to provide diet and nutrition counseling as well as developing collaborative care models to deliver nutrition advice will reduce the health and economic burden of atherosclerotic cardiovascular disease to a degree not previously recognized." It goes on to note that "despite evidence that physicians are willing to undertake this task and are seen as credible sources of diet information, they engage patients in diet counseling at less than desirable rates and cite insufficient nutrition knowledge and training as barriers to carrying out this role … These data align with ongoing evidence of large and persistent gaps in medical nutrition education and training in the United States … "

The American Family Physician journal is getting on board as well. The June 1, 2018 edition contained an article titled "Diets for Health: Goals and Guidelines," which reviewed the pros and cons of various diets that are touted as being healthy. The article points out that plant proteins are preferable, and cites the health benefits of fruits and vegetables, legumes (beans, lentils, chick peas), whole grains, healthy fats, and spices.

In a high-lighted box titled "What is New on This Topic: Diets For Health," the article notes:

- "Large, prospective cohort studies show that vegetarian diets reduce the risk of coronary heart disease and type 2 diabetes mellitus, and that vegan diets offer additional benefits for obesity, hypertension, type 2 diabetes, and cardio-vascular disease."
- "Eating nuts, including peanuts, is associated with decreased cardiovascular disease and mortality, lower body weight, and lower diabetes risk."
- "In a prospective cohort study, consumption of artificially sweetened beverages increased the risk of type 2 diabetes … "

Of course, Drs. Esselstyn, Fuhrman, Greger, McDougall, Barnard and others have been telling us these things for years; this information really isn't new. What's new is that the medical establishment is finally listening.

At my fiftieth medical school reunion in Denver, graduating medical students told me they still aren't being taught much about nutrition or prevention. But maybe this will finally change, and in the near future medical students will learn that health isn't all about pills and procedure—that inexpensive, low-tech lifestyle changes can prevent and reverse many of the chronic, costly diseases that afflict so many Americans.

"When I was 88 years old, I gave up meat entirely
and switched to a plant foods diet following a slight stroke.
During the following months, I not only lost 50 pounds,
but gained strength in my legs and picked up stamina.
Now, at age 93, I'm on the same plant-based diet,
and I still don't eat any meat or dairy products.
I either swim, walk, or paddle a canoe daily
and I feel the best I've felt since my heart problems began."

– Dr. Benjamin Spock

ADVANCES IN HEALTH CARE ARE NOT ALL ABOUT GLITTER AND EXPENSE

On August 1, 2017 there was a front-page article in the *Denver Post* with the heading "U.S. hospitals set record for fast heart attack care." This referred to opening up an acutely clogged artery with a stent, fast enough to save heart muscle and lives. This of course is good news, because heart attacks are the main cause of death in America.

However, this high-tech solution is an example of how, in modern American society, people are looking for sexy, expensive, headline-grabbing technology to solve their health problems. At least 25 percent of heart attack (myocardial infarction) victims die suddenly, before they can dial 911. The good news is that almost all heart attacks can be prevented. If patients take personal responsibility for their health by exercising and eating an optimal diet, and if primary care physicians do their job, there should be no need for stents. Furthermore, lifestyle modification is cheap and doesn't have side effects. But this approach doesn't get much press, or much attention in medical school.

We hear about genomics eventually being the answer to many health problems. However, as Robert Pearl, M.D. says in his book *Mistreated,* "The promise of genomic medicine has yet to be fulfilled, and probably won't be for years, if ever." He notes that "everyone would be better off eating healthier foods, exercising regularly, and getting the appropriate prevention screenings." He also points out that "extending the full benefits of immunization to every person worldwide by 2020 would prevent an estimated 20 million deaths—mostly in children—and untold suffering from blindness, paralysis, and deafness for millions more."

The health tip on Medical Devices talked about robotic surgery. The robots are expensive, robotic surgery takes longer than conventional surgery, and patient outcomes are no better than with traditional surgery. However, due to marketing, patients think robotic surgery is the way to go, so hospitals buy this expensive technology and urologists use it.

Seatbelts are low tech and inexpensive, but save more than 15,000 lives every year in the U.S.

One of the greatest advances in health care in the last 100 years was improving the way doctors organize their thoughts and medical records when they see patients.

HEALTH CARE SYSTEM—PROBLEMS WITH

When I was in medical school in the 1960s, a patient would come in with say hypertension, diabetes, back pain, and a cold. The note would often intermingle all the problems in one paragraph, with no clear diagnosis or plan for each problem. In the late 1960s, Dr. Lawrence Weed, at the University of Vermont, changed this with the problem oriented medical record and SOAP notes. SOAP is an acronym for subjective complaints (what the patient tells the doctor); objective (what the doctor finds on exam and lab and other studies); assessment (what the doctor thinks the diagnosis is including other possibilities); and plan (what the doctor's plan of treatment is). Today, thanks to Dr. Weed, each patient record now has a list of the permanent problems such as hypertension, diabetes, chronic back pain; and a SOAP note should be present (it doesn't always happen) for each problem a patient presents with at a particular visit. This forces doctors to think in a logical fashion about each problem. This simple, low-tech approach standardized doctors' practices and record keeping and improved quality of care as much as any high tech development in the twentieth century.

The point is when it comes to health care, all the glitter is not gold, and some of the most important medical advances in modern medicine have been inexpensive and low-tech.

"The world's strongest animals are plant eaters.
Gorillas, Buffaloes, Elephants and me."

– Patrik Baboumian,
German stongman competitor

HEARING LOSS CAN LEAD
TO MULTIPLE HEALTH PROBLEMS

The cochlea is a sea shell-shaped structure in the inner ear (inside the skull) that converts sound vibrations to nerve signals that are transmitted to the brain. The brain then "decodes" the signals, resulting in what we experience as sound. There are several causes of hearing loss, including congenital abnormalities and side effects from drugs such as certain antibiotics. The most common cause of hearing loss is damage to the cochlea as we age.

Although age-related hearing loss is common, not everybody gets it, so it isn't "normal." Risk factors for age-related hearing loss are: exposure to loud noises, male sex, smoking, diabetes, central obesity (heaviness around the middle), atherosclerosis (hardening of the arteries), chronic inflammation, untreated high blood pressure, and poor diet.

The most important cause of hearing loss, and the easiest to prevent, is exposure to loud noises. According to *Nutrition Action,* published by the Center For Science In The Public Interest, "Prolonged exposure to any noise at or above 85 decibels can cause gradual hearing loss." Examples of noises in the safe range are: whisper, 30 decibels; refrigerator 40, normal conversation 60, dishwasher 75. Examples of sounds above the safe range are: heavy city traffic, school cafeteria 85 decibels; power mower 90; wood-shop, snowmobile 100; personal stereo at maximum level 105; rock concert 110; ambulance siren 120; jet taking off 140; firecracker, shotgun firing 140–165.

Hearing loss can lead to poor quality of life, and specifically the following problems:

- Relationship issues, especially with your spouse or significant other
- Loneliness
- Depression and anxiety
- Accidents (e.g. not hearing a car that is backing up or a biker on the bike path)
- Of most concern is cognitive decline and dementia (which makes sense because hearing loss results in less brain stimulation)

Treatment of hearing loss has been shown to prevent these problems. According to the CDC, 20 percent of adults ages 40 to 69 and 43 percent of those over 70 have hearing loss. Age-related loss usually presents as inability to hear high-frequency tones (such as your wife if you're a married man), sometimes associated with tinnitus (ringing in the ears). Unfortunately, only 1 in 7 Americans with hearing loss is being treated with hearing aids.

If you or other people think you have hearing loss, don't be in denial. See your PCP or an audiologist (hearing specialist) for a test; or take a 5 dollar online test by going to *nationalhearingtest.org* (you need a quiet room and a land line). The problem with hearing aids is that they typically cost at least $2,500 per ear, although people say they are less expensive at Costco. Medicare doesn't pay for them, (although now that we know the health problems that result for hearing loss, they should). Another option is assisted listening devices (ALDs). These devices amplify sound, and are a few hundred dollars rather than thousands. However, some brands can make hearing worse. The University of California, Berkeley, *Wellness Letter* suggests the following websites to help find a good ALD: *tinyurl.com/ALD-NAD, tinyurl.com/RERC-hear,* and *tinyurl.com/ALD-NIH.* Audiologists can also help you, but are sometimes biased if they sell hearing aids.

Due to government regulations, job-related hearing loss is much less common than it once was. The best thing you can do to prevent hearing loss is to avoid loud noises, and if you can't, wear ear protection (e.g. while mowing the lawn and using power tools).

HEARING LOSS

*"Nothing will benefit human health
and increase the chances for survival of life on Earth
as much as the evolution to a vegetarian diet."*

– Albert Einstein

GET YOUR FLU SHOT

The Center for Disease Control (CDC) recommends that everyone over the age of 6 months get a flu shot by the end of October. Children under the age of 6 months should not receive flu shots, so it's particularly important that these children's care givers are immunized. Children 6 months and older need 2 flu shots, 4 weeks apart. During the 2016–2017 flu season, there were 77 deaths in children that probably would have been prevented had they received flu shots.

Adults need just 1 shot, and people 65 years and older need an extra-strength shot. The 1918 Spanish flu epidemic resulted in 675,000 American deaths. About 48,000 deaths occurred during the 2003–2004 flu season. Of lesser concern but still important is that influenza accounts for many days of lost work and school absences.

Influenza is caused by viruses. The most severe forms are influenza A and B, with C being a milder disease. In temperate climates, the flu viruses are usually active during the colder, late fall, winter and early spring months. It takes several days for the shots to "kick in." Flu shots can be obtained in most doctors' offices, in pharmacies, and at public health offices. Due to changes in the genetic makeup of the flu viruses from year-to-year, called "genetic drift," the makeup of the flu vaccine changes each year. Allergy to egg is not a contraindication to getting the shot, although if you have an egg allergy you should mention it to whoever is vaccinating you.

Side effects, other than mild soreness for a day or two where the shot was given, are rare. People sometimes say that the flu shot gave them the flu, but that has never been proven to occur. The average adult gets 5, non-flu viral infections a year such as colds, so out of the millions of flu shots that are given every year some people will co-incidentally come down with one of these other viral infections and blame it on the flu shot they just had.

Influenza is highly contagious, and is transmitted by the respiratory route, meaning nasal discharge and coughing. The incubation period is 1–4 days. Typical symptoms include fever, chills, malaise (feeling really crummy), generalized aching, chest discomfort, headache, nasal stuffiness, dry cough, and sore throat. Elderly patients often present with lassitude and confusion but not the other symptoms. Frequent flu complications include sinus and ear infections, bronchitis and pneumonia (viral and bacterial), with pneumonia usually being the cause of flu-related deaths. Young children taking aspirin can develop Reye syndrome, which affects the liver and brain and can lead to death.

Did you know that a timely flu shot can reduce cardiovascular mortality (heart attacks and stroke) by 50 percent? Bacterial and viral infections such as influenza can cause inflammation that can trigger rupture of arterial plaque, the cause of heart attacks and strokes. According to Bale and Doneen in their book *Beat the Heart Attack Gene,* a large study showed that up to 91,000 Americans die annually from heart attacks and strokes triggered by the flu, and these are not included in the statistics noted above for flu-related deaths.

Rapid flu tests done in doctors' offices are helpful in diagnosis, although false positives and negatives can occur. Remember that flu shots only prevent influenza A and B, but not colds or stomach or intestinal flu. They are not 100 percent effective in preventing influenza, but the disease tends to be shorter and milder in people who have been immunized. So be proactive about your health, and get the flu shot if you haven't already.

IMMUNIZATIONS

"I don't understand why asking people to eat a well-balanced vegetarian diet is considered drastic, while it is medically conservative to cut people open and put them on cholesterol lowering drugs for the rest of their lives."

– Dean Ornish, M.D.

THE "PNEUMONIA SHOT" CAN PREVENT SERIOUS ILLNESS AND DEATH

Pneumococcal bacteria are present as part of the normal bacterial microbiome of the nose in many children and adults. However, in certain circumstances, such as when the body is weakened by influenza or other viral upper respiratory infections, pneumococci can cause serious and sometimes fatal illnesses, including the following:

- Pneumonia, which even in the age of antibiotics still kills people
- Meningitis, which can cause permanent neurological damage and death
- Sepsis, which is an overwhelming blood infection that is often fatal
- Bone and joint infections
- Ear and sinus infections

Certain conditions can make people more susceptible to severe pneumococcal infections:

- Very young and old age, particularly age less than 2 in children and over 64 in adults
- Absence of a spleen, usually due to trauma
- Chronic heart, liver and kidney disease; diabetes; asthma and emphysema
- Weakened immune system that occurs with conditions such as cancer being treated with chemotherapy; HIV/AIDS; alcoholism
- Medications that weaken the immune system such as long-term cortisone
- Blood disorders such as sickle cell disease
- Cochlear implants
- Smoking

There are several sub-types of pneumococcal bacteria. A few decades ago, vaccines were developed that are effective against many of these sub-types. Although the vaccines are not 100 percent effective, immunized people who develop pneumococcal disease usually have less severe disease, with shorter courses, compared with non-immunized people.

PCV13 vaccine (brand name Prevenar) is given to children at ages 2, 4, 6, and 12–15 months of age. Children age 6 through 18 and adults age 19 to 65 should also be given the PCV13 if they have any of the risk factors listed in the second paragraph. All adults age 65 and older should also receive the PCV13.

Another pneumococcal vaccine, called PPSV23 (brand name Pneumovax), should be given to all adults 65 and older; and to adults younger than 65 if they have any of the conditions listed in paragraph 2.

Pneumonia shots can be obtained in most doctors' offices, most pharmacies, and county public health offices. It takes 2–3 weeks for them to "kick in." Side effects other than minor aching around the injection site are rare.

The bottom line is that to prevent serious illness and death from pneumococcal infections, and to prevent less serious illness such as pneumococcal ear and sinus infections: (1) All children should receive 4 doses of PCV13. (2) All adults 65 and older should receive PCV13 and the PPSV23 (Pneumovax), although not at the same visit. (3) Adults under 65 and with conditions listed above, or who have children with these conditions, should check with their healthcare provider or a public health nurse for recommendations. This information is also provided by the CDC (Center for Disease Control) on the Internet.

"For both optimal health and weight loss, you must consume a diet with a high nutrient-per-calorie ratio."

– Joel Fuhrman, M.D.

IMMUNIZATIONS

THE IMMUNIZATION SUCCESS STORY

It's been said that America doesn't have a health care system, but instead we have an expensive disease management system; we wait until preventable diseases occur and then spend billions of dollars managing them. There is one shining example of how our system should work: immunizations, which save millions of lives, prevent millions of cases of disability (e.g. deafness from measles, birth defects from Rubella), and save the health care system billions of dollars. The previous tip discussed the "pneumonia shot," and before that the flu shot, and how these immunizations prevent serious disease and death.

Vaccine, used for immunization, is defined as "a suspension of attenuated or killed microorganisms (bacteria, viruses, or rickettsia), or of antigenic proteins derived from them, administered for the prevention, amelioration, or treatments of infectious diseases." In other words, vaccines mobilize our natural defense mechanisms, resulting in antibodies that prevent disease, without causing us to experience the disease. In underdeveloped countries, infectious diseases are still a major cause of death and disability, and this was once true in our country, but immunizations changed that.

In 1900, there were 21,064 cases of smallpox in the U.S., with 894 deaths. In 1920, there were 469,924 measles cases and 7,575 deaths. In 1920, there were 147,991 cases of diphtheria, with 13,170 deaths. In 1922, there were 107,473 cases of pertussis (whooping cough) with 5,099 deaths. From 1951 to 1954, there was an average of 16,316 cases of paralytic polio per year with 1879 deaths. Prior to introduction in 1987 of the Hib vaccine against the Hemophilus bacteria, there were 20,000 cases of childhood infection a year, causing meningitis and mental retardation and many deaths. Since vaccines were introduced for these and other diseases, they have almost disappeared in the U.S. There has not been a case of polio in the U.S. since 1979, and smallpox was eradicated worldwide in 1977.

There are two vaccines that prevent cancer: one is the HPV vaccine, which prevents the sexually transmitted wart virus that is the cause of cancer of the cervix and and which can also cause cancer of the mouth and throat via oral sex transmission. The other is hepatitis B vaccine, because chronic hepatitis B causes liver cancer.

Are vaccines safe? The short answer is yes, extremely safe. Minor irritation at the injection site is common with many types of immunizations. Children can experience post-immunization irritability and fever, but these symptoms are less common since the introduction of the acellular pertussis vaccine (part of the DPT shot). Serious side effects from vaccines, such as anaphylactic allergic reactions, have an incidence of approximately one per 1 million vaccine doses, and can usually be successfully treated. I tell patients that getting immunized is like wearing seat belts: very rarely someone drowns in a car accident when their car goes into a river and they can't get their seat belt off, but almost always it's safest to wear seatbelts.

Unfortunately, there is a small but vociferous group of people, including some alternative providers, who make unfounded claims on the internet and elsewhere about alleged harm from vaccinations. Several years ago, a British scientist wrote a paper claiming a link between autism and the MMR (measles, mumps, rubella or German measles) vaccine. His paper was later found to be a hoax, and multiple subsequent studies have failed to show such a link. However, it has taken time to educate the public about the truth.

I recall in the 1950s lining up to get the polio vaccine, and my relief and other parents' relief that our kids would never come down with dreaded paralytic polio. As a freshman medical student in Denver in 1964, I looked in a room at Colorado General Hospital that was filled with iron lung machines used for patients who were completely paralyzed by polio and who therefore couldn't breathe. This was a few years after essentially everyone in the U.S. had been immunized against polio, so these machines were no longer needed. There are multiple infectious diseases that we no longer have to worry about because of the success of immunization programs in this country. If we travel to underdeveloped countries, especially in the tropics, we can get immunized against infectious diseases that are still prevalent there, such as cholera and yellow fever. And thanks to the WHO (World Health Organization), many people in underdeveloped countries are getting immunized. In his book *Mistreated*, Dr. Robert Pearl says that "extending the full benefits of immunization to every person worldwide by 2020 would prevent an estimated 20 million deaths—mostly in children—and untold suffering from blindness, paralysis, and deafness for millions more."

To see if you or your child are up to date on immunizations, check with your primary care provider, the CDC (Center for Disease Control) website, or at a county public health office.

IMMUNIZATIONS

EAT FRUIT AND VEGETABLES TO AVOID BLINDNESS FROM MACULAR DEGENERATION

Most of us want to live a long life, as long as we maintain a life of good quality. This includes keeping our vision intact (and our mind).

In developed countries, age-related macular degeneration (ARMD) is the leading cause of blindness in people 55 and older. It currently affects 11 million Americans and by 2020 it is expected to affect 20 million. Thirty percent of Americans over the age of 75 have it. There are two types of ARMD, wet and dry. Although treatment can slow the progression of visual loss, there is no cure for ARMD.

The retina is located in the back of the eye. The central portion of the retina is called the macula, and is responsible for detailed vision and central vision (as opposed to peripheral vision). The human eye is a good example of how over millions of years, humans evolved to eat plants. On his website *nutritionfacts.org*, Dr. Michael Greger notes that dietary yellow plant pigments called carotenoids are taken up by the retina. These pigments absorb blue light and protect the retina from sun damage. If diet doesn't contain enough carotenoids, the retina is damaged, leading to macular degeneration.

Risk factors for developing ARMD are age, family history, certain genetic abnormalities, smoking, obesity, high blood pressure, high cholesterol, and a diet deficient in fruit and vegetables. In his book *Eat to Live*, Joel Fuhrman, M.D. notes that "low carotenoid levels in the macula are now considered a risk factor for macular degeneration" and that "if you eat greens at least 5 times per week, your risk drops by more than 86 percent."

Lutein and zeaxanthin are two of the carotenoids that are most important in promoting eye health. Here are some examples of micrograms of these phyto (plant) nutrients certain foods contain:

- One cup cooked kale, 28,470 micrograms
- One cup cooked spinach, 27,710
- One cup cooked red bell pepper, 13,600

The egg industry advertises that eggs are a good source of these carotenoids, and eggs do contain some, depending on what the chickens they came from ate. But in reality, the amount eggs contain is minimal. For example, goji berries contain 60 times more than eggs do.

When ophthalmologists diagnose ARMD, they often prescribe pills containing vitamin C, beta-carotene, E, zinc, copper, lutein, and zeaxanthin. You certainly want to follow your doctor's advice if you have a disease like this that can lead to blindness. But you want to do everything you can to stack the deck in your favor by also eating a variety of fruit and vegetables.

Diabetic retinopathy is another top cause of blindness in developed countries. Type 2 diabetes can be prevented—and if caught early enough, reversed—by a plant-based diet. And Dr. Walter Kempner proved in the 1930s that diabetic retinopathy can be reversed with plant-based nutrition.

MACULAR DEGNERATION

"Don't let perfect be the enemy of good."

– Voltaire, French Enlightenment philosopher

(Don't drive yourself crazy by spending all day in the grocery store reading food labels, looking for the perfect food.)

COULD THE BACTERIA IN YOUR GUT BE MAKING YOU FAT?

One of the new frontiers in medicine is the gut microbiome. This refers to the microorganisms that inhabit the human gut, which consists primarily of bacteria, but also includes viruses, and fungi such as yeast. This health tip is about gut bacteria, which are at least three times greater in number than all the cells in the human body.

Scientists are finding more and more links between the type of bacteria we have in our gastrointestinal tracts—particularly our colons—and various aspects of our health. An issue of the University of California, Berkeley, *Wellness Letter* contains an article by John Swartzberg, M.D., chair of the editorial board, about antibiotics and obesity. He points out that research "has found that the composition of the microbiome can influence energy metabolism as well as how carbohydrates and fats are digested, thus affecting the risk of obesity."

One of the reasons livestock are treated with antibiotics is that they cause animals to gain weight. In humans, studies have shown that "impoverished, malnourished children who are treated with antibiotics gain weight." A group of intestinal bacteria called Firmicules "cause us to absorb more calories from the same amount of food" compared with another group called Bacteroidetes. Therefore, a preponderance of Firmicules is associated with obesity, and a preponderance of Bacteroidetes is associated with being lean.

One factor that can affect our microbiome is what we eat. Our gut bacteria thrive on fiber and resistant (indigestible) starch. Fiber is found in plants, but not in animal products. People who eat a purely plant-based diet have gut bacteria that promote being lean. People on an animal-based diet have gut bacteria that promote obesity, and many chronic diseases including cardiovascular disease and diabetes.

The microbiome can also be affected by antibiotics. Although antibiotics can be life-saving when used to treat severe infectious diseases such as meningitis and bacterial pneumonia, they are over-prescribed by doctors, and patients often demand them for minor illnesses. According to Dr. Swartzberg, even a short course of antibiotics can affect the gut flora for up to a year. A study reported in the *JAMA Pediatrics* journal "found that children who took antibiotics—especially broad spectrum antibiotics—at least four times before age two had an elevated risk of becoming obese by age five." There is even a link between antibiotics given in the second and third trimester of pregnancy and having offspring who become obese.

In conclusion, you will be more apt to attain and maintain an ideal body weight if you have a health-promoting gut microbiome, and the way to achieve that is to eat a plant-based diet, and avoid antibiotics unless absolutely necessary. If you continue to eat animal products, try to avoid meat that contains antibiotics.

MICROBIOME

"Having the USDA design your food pyramid
is like having Al Capone do your taxes."

– Caldwell Esselstyn, M.D.

HOW MINDFULNESS MEDITATION CAN IMPROVE YOUR EMOTIONAL AND PHYSICAL HEALTH

Stress is harmful to our emotional as well as our physical health. There is now a large body of scientific evidence supporting the mind-body connection. As Dean Ornish, M.D. points out in his most recent book *The Spectrum,* "Stress can suppress your immune function, cause a heart attack or stroke, increase your risk of cancer, delay wound healing, promote inflammation, cause you to gain weight, impair your memory, cause depression, exacerbate diabetes, and worsen your sexual function. Just for starters." Stress can also damage your DNA, which contributes to aging.

How does stress do all this? It initiates the "fight-or-flight" response: stress hormones such as cortisol are released, muscles contract, blood pressure rises, blood clots more easily, arteries constrict, neurotransmitters in the brain such as serotonin are affected, sleep is disrupted, and often anxiety and depression ensue.

So, stress affects our emotions, thoughts, and bodies, but what many people don't know is that we can control our thoughts, thereby preventing this harmful cascade. We all have constant chatter going on in our minds, and—particularly in people prone to depression and anxiety—many of these thoughts are repetitive (i.e. obsessive) and negative. This chatter prevents us from being mindful (focused) about a lot of what we do every day, including eating.

If you are under stress, and most of us are to one degree or another, consider a class in mindfulness meditation. You will learn how to sit in a relaxed position, how to focus on your breathing, and how to control your brain chatter—particularly the negative and obsessive thoughts. If you practice mindfulness meditation every day, ideally first thing in the morning, you will find that you feel much more centered the rest of the day, that you are more positive and more focused, and that your mood improves. As a result, you will be less prone to anxiety and depression, and your physical health will benefit as well.

Dr. Ornish proved 25 years ago that heart disease can be reversed with exercise and a plant-based, whole food, low-fat diet. As he became more aware of the mind-body connection, he added stress reduction to his program, which is now approved by Medicare. His book *The Spectrum* includes a chapter about "the stress-management spectrum" in which he recommends mindfulness meditation.

You can find mindfulness meditation programs on the Internet. The Mindful Life Program is a national foundation and hosts a periodic "Foundations of Mindfulness" course taught by Laura Bartels in Carbondale, Colorado (*mindfullifeprogram.org*). The brochure reads as follows: "Combine meditation training with practical, accessible, and universal skills that empower you to engage in your life with attention and intention. Learn to experience life's events consciously and be able to respond with clarity and wisdom. Transform your life and cultivate genuine, lasting happiness."

You can also read John Bruna's (founder of The Mindful Life Program and former Buddhist monk) book called *The Wisdom of a Meaningful Life: The Essence of Mindfulness*.

To some, this might sound like a new-age fad. But it is actually ancient, having been practiced by Christian monks as well as Eastern religious disciples for centuries.

MINDFULNESS MEDITATION

"Cows' milk protein may be the
single most significant chemical carcinogen
to which humans are exposed."

- T. Colin Campbell, PhD

HEALTH PROBLEMS ASSOCIATED WITH BEING OVERWEIGHT

Obesity is becoming more prevalent every year in America, and as we export our diet to the rest of the world, obesity is increasing world-wide. The body mass index (BMI) is used to define obesity, with normal BMI being 18.5–24.9, overweight being 25–29.9, and obesity being greater than 30. This measurement is calculated by dividing body weight in kilograms by height in meters squared, and if you want to see what your BMI is, calculators can be found on the Internet.

However, BMI is not a perfect measurement of a person's risk for health problems from adipose tissue (fat):

- Irrespective of BMI, if waist circumference measured just above your hip bones (about the level of your navel) is 35 inches or greater in a female or 40 inches or greater in a male (lower cutoff in Asians and East Indians), then harmful visceral fat is present—fat in and around your internal organs.
- If you look at your naked profile in the mirror and you have even a small "belly," you have visceral fat, even if your BMI is in the normal range.
- Weight gain is common as we age in this country but it isn't normal. If you are around 50 or older, you should weigh what you did when you graduated from high school (this rule can't be used for younger people because so many of them are overweight now).
- If you go from a BMI of 18 to a BMI of 24, both of which are in the normal range, this represents a 40-pound weight gain, and even a five pound weight gain is associated with disease.

Here are some of the health problems associated with being overweight:
- Increased incidence of heart attacks, the main cause of death in the U.S.
- Increased incidence of strokes (another common cause of death and a major cause of disability)
- High blood pressure
- Increased risk of diabetes (which commonly results in complications such as loss of vision, cardiovascular disease, kidney failure and nerve damage)

- Increased risk of obstructive sleep apnea
- Increased risk of GERD (gastroesophageal reflux disease)
- Increased risk of several types of cancer: breast, uterus, pancreas, kidney, colon and rectum, esophagus
- Mobility problems including degenerative arthritis of hips and knees
- Gall bladder disease
- Chronic, low-grade inflammation

In summary, gaining weight in Americans as they age is common but is not normal, and contributes to several health problems.

"As a physician,
I am embarrassed by my profession's
lack of interest in healthier lifestyles.
We need to change the way we approach chronic disease."

– Caldwell Esselstyn, M.D.

HOW TO ACHIEVE AND MAINTAIN IDEAL BODY WEIGHT

Weight loss in this country is a multi-billion-dollar industry, and there are many diets out there, some of which work short-term. However, if you look at the research that's been done on different diets, the only thing that works long-term is not a "diet," but rather a lifestyle modification: regular exercise and consumption of plant-based, whole (unprocessed) food diet with no salt, sugar, or added oil. If you adopt the following tips, you will achieve your ideal body weight; and if you follow them the rest of your life, you will maintain it. A side benefit is that you will also achieve optimal health:

- Avoid calorie-dense food, which includes meat, seafood, dairy, eggs, sugar (read food labels—4 grams of sugar is a teaspoon), added vegetable oil (120 calories per tablespoon), and processed food.
- Substitute foods that are low in calorie density but high in nutrients—fruit, vegetables, and whole grains (if the total carb:fiber ratio on the food label is 5:1 or less, the product has lots of fiber and whole grains).
- Don't skip meals, especially breakfast.
- Chew your food rather than drink it.
- Eat slowly and mindfully. Italian actress Sofia Loren once said that "the reason Americans are overweight is that they don't enjoy their food enough." Consider eating with chopsticks.
- Eat high-fiber food, which fills you up without giving you lots of calories. Plants have fiber, animal products don't.
- Eat food that feeds the health-promoting bacteria in your gut, particularly the bacteria that help regulate your metabolism—that would be plants.
- Avoid addictive food: salt, sugar, and fat. Big Food is shameless about adding these things to their products.
- Although what you don't eat is much more important for weight loss than exercise, the latter is important for weight maintenance. Exercise hard enough so you could talk but not sing, for at least 30 minutes a day.
- If you have a sit-down job, get up and move around every 30 minutes, and/or use a standup desk.

- If you watch a lot of TV, get up periodically or buy a small device that you can pedal to put in front of your TV chair.

For more information, a good book to read is *The End of Dieting,* by Joel Fuhrman, M.D. Good plant-based cookbooks include *Oh She Glows* (some of the recipes call for oil—substitute ground flaxseed and/or unsweetened apple sauce), *Forks Over Knives Cookbook, Isa Does It, Thug Kitchen, Simply Delicious, Vegan Richa's Indian Kitchen,* and *How Not to Die Cookbook.*

"More people die because of the way they eat
than by tobacco use, accidents or any
other lifestyle or environmental factor."

– T. Colin Campbell, PhD

OBESITY

HOW NOT TO DIE FROM PARKINSON'S DISEASE

Parkinson's is the second most common degenerative brain disease, after Alzheimer's. It affects 1 percent of the population, with around 60,000 new cases in the U.S. every year—mainly people over 55. Men and women are affected equally, as are all ethnic groups. The disease is slowly progressive, and typical symptoms include tremor, rigidity, and difficulty initiating movement such as getting up from a chair and walking. Depression and cognitive impairment are common.

Head trauma can result in Parkinson's, so the disease is relatively common in boxers (remember Mohammad Ali?) and football players. Some people have a genetic propensity to develop the disease, but as is the case with so many diseases, environment determines whether or not these genes are activated. So what can you change in your environment to protect against Parkinson's?

Dr. Michael Greger in his book *How Not to Die* has a chapter about Parkinson's, and his website *nutritionfacts.org* contains additional information. Dr. Greger presents compelling evidence that most cases of Parkinson's are linked to environmental pollutants, many of which are neurotoxic (damage the brain and sometimes other parts of the nervous system). Some of these harmful chemicals are:

- Arsenic—the primary source is poultry
- Mercury—the primary source is fish
- DDT, which has been banned but it still found in meat
- PCBs, which have also been banned but are still found in fish, fish oil, eggs, dairy (especially cheese), and meat
- Dioxins which accumulate in the fat of animals including chickens, in eggs, and in farm-raised catfish

Unfortunately, these toxic chemicals are ubiquitous in our environment and in our bodies, and contribute not only to Parkinson's but to many other diseases, including cancer. Dr. Greger notes that the CDC measures levels of chemical pollutants in thousands of Americans every few years, and for example has found that "the bodies of most women in the United States are contaminated with heavy metals, toxic solvents, endocrine disrupting chemicals, fire retardants, chemicals from plastics, polychlorinated biphenyls (PCPs) and … DDT." Men have even higher levels of some pollutants than women, and children from neonates on up are affected as well (e.g. DDT is detected in 95 percent of umbilical cord blood samples taken at birth).

What can we do to lessen our contact with toxins, and thereby lower our risk for Parkinson's and the other diseases that have links to these toxins? It certainly helps if you buy organic, although organic often costs more and isn't necessary if you're buying something with a thick skin or peel, such as an orange, banana, or avocado. By far the most effective action you can take, though, is to eat at the bottom of the food chain by eating only plant-based food. For example, a cow may eat 75,000 pounds' worth of plants before being slaughtered for meat, and even if the cow is raised on an organic farm, pollutants blow in from adjacent farms and come down in rain. These chemicals are stored in the cows' meat and fat. When you eat meat you get 14 times, and dairy 5.5 times, the pollutants than if you just ate plants, at the bottom of the food chain.

It's interesting that nicotine has neuroprotective effects, and smokers have a 50 percent lower incidence of Parkinson's. Tobacco is in the nightshade family of vegetables, and you can get the same neuroprotective effects, without the many harmful effects of smoking, by eating other nightshade plants: tomatoes, potatoes, eggplant, and peppers.

Caffeine in coffee and tea is associated with a 1/3 lower risk of Parkinson's. Drinking 2 cups of coffee, 4 cups of black tea, or 8 cups of green tea a day improves symptoms of Parkinson's. Uric acid is neuroprotective, and low levels are associated with increased Parkinson's risk. High levels, though, cause gout, kidney, and heart disease. The sweet spot seems to be a level of 5 to 7. Drinking cows' milk lowers uric acid, which may be another reason (besides environmental toxins) that dairy is linked to Parkinson's.

"There is absolutely no nutrient, no protein, no vitamin, no mineral that can't be obtained from plant-based foods."

— Michael Klapper, M.D.

DO YOU REALLY NEED THAT CT SCAN?

An issue of the University of California, Berkeley *Wellness Letter* contained an important article: "Should You Worry About CT Scans?" X-rays were invented some 120 years ago, and they clearly improved doctors' diagnostic capability. CT scans were invented in the 1970s, and improved diagnostic capability considerably more. I can't imagine practicing medicine in the days before X-rays were available, but was in training in the 1960s and early 1970s, before CTs. Both of these imaging techniques were a boon to both patients and doctors.

However, there are downsides to this technology, the most serious one being radiation exposure, cost being another. Soon after X-rays were in common use, they were found to cause hair loss and burns in patients and in personnel who performed them. In spite of that, X-rays were used for conditions such as enlarged tonsils. And those of us my age (born in 1941) recall going to a Buster Brown shoe store and putting our feet in a fluoroscopic X-ray machine to determine shoe fit. After decades, the seriousness of radiation exposure became apparent and protection was offered to patients, doctors, and techs. We now know that radiation causes dangerous free-radicals and cancer-causing DNA damage.

CT stands for computed tomography. These scans create several cross-sectional images, and involve many times more radiation than simple X-rays. CT scans are used to diagnose conditions such as heart disease, cancer, the cause of abdominal and pelvic pain, kidney stones, and injuries. According to the Berkeley article, "CT scans of the abdomen and pelvis tend to produce the most radiation, averaging 100 to 200 times more than a simple chest X-ray, 1,500 times more than dental X-rays, and 200,000 times more than airport scanners." Other types of imaging that utilize high levels of radiation include cardiac stress tests with nuclear imaging, fluoroscopy, and PET scans.

Radiation is cumulative over a lifetime, and is particularly damaging to infants and children, even more so to the fetus. Radiation from diagnostic studies is thought to cause about 2 percent of new cancer cases in the U.S. A paper published in a respected medical journal in 2009 claimed that CT scans done in 2007 were projected to cause 29,000 extra cases of cancer and eventually 14,500 deaths. Unfortunately, Americans are exposed to at least 6 times more radiation from medical imaging (mostly CT) than

RADIATION EXPOSURE IN MEDICINE

we were three decades ago. According to the Berkeley *Wellness Letter,* it's thought that 1/3 to 1/2 of CT scans may be unnecessary.

According to Consumer Reports, here are the factors that contribute to overuse of CT scans:

- Financial incentives: We have a healthcare system that rewards providers for ordering lots of tests. Some physicians and most hospitals own radiology equipment or diagnostic centers—when CT is easily available it's used.
- Fear of lawsuits, which may account for 35 percent of diagnostic imaging.
- Uninformed physicians, who don't understand the amount of radiation CT scans cause, the dangers associated with that radiation, or that other types radiation-free imaging such as ultrasound and MRI may be just as adequate.
- Misinformed patients: Fewer than 1 in 6 patients in a Consumer Reports survey said their doctors had warned them about radiation risks or that there were safer alternatives.
- Patient demand: Many patients insist on an X-ray or CT scan.
- Lack of regulation: Unlike mammography, there are no federal radiation limits or universal standards for CT imaging.

What can you do? Here's what Consumer Report and the Berkeley *Wellness Letter* recommend:

- Ask if the CT scan is really necessary, will improve your health, and if a radiation-free alternative is an option.
- Check credentials for the imaging facility and the tech.
- Get the right dose for your size. The smaller and thinner you are, the lower the radiation dose you need. Children require much smaller doses but according to Consumer Reports they are often given adult doses.
- Ask for the lowest effective dose, make sure the scan is limited to the body part in question and that adjacent areas are shielded.
- The radiation dose of a CT scan can vary even within the same hospital, and a 2013 JAMA Pediatrics study claimed that decreasing the highest doses could cut in half the number of future radiation-related cancers.
- If the recommended CT scan is a repeat of a previous one you've had, ask why it needs to be repeated.
- Ask your doctor if they have a financial interest in the CT scanner, and if so, get a second opinion.
- Avoid total body scans, which often result in what doctors call "incidentalomas." A scan shows a small shadow, which almost always is an incidental finding of no significance, but to be 100 percent certain instead of 99.9 percent, additional imaging and even biopsies are ordered.

RADIATION EXPOSURE IN MEDICINE

• Avoid cone-beam CT dental X-rays, especially in children.

Remember that in many cases, CT scans are appropriate and necessary and can be life-saving. But they should be used with caution, and your provider is obligated to discuss the pros and cons and alternative options. If you do need a scan but will have a large out-of-pocket expense, check prices at different facilities.

"Although scientists can often be as
resistant to new ideas as anyone,
the process of science ensures that,
over time, good ideas and theories prevail."

– Dean Ornish, M.D.

RADIATION EXPOSURE IN MEDICINE

AN UNDER-APPRECIATED BUT SERIOUS CONDITION: CENTRAL SLEEP APNEA

Apnea refers to absent breathing. Sleep apnea refers to periods of absent breathing during sleep. Obstructive sleep apnea (OSA) is the most common form of sleep apnea, affecting about 18 million Americans, 90 percent of whom are undiagnosed. Most, although not all, people with OSA snore, and often their bed partners notice several seconds of absent breathing followed by a loud snort. Breathing effort continues during the apnea but airflow is prevented due to blockage of the upper air passages in the mouth and throat due to conditions such as enlarged tonsils and adenoids in kids, and obesity or receding chin in adults. Most people with OSA aren't aware they have a problem, but often complain of not feeling rested when they awaken in the morning, and feeling sleepy during the day.

The second type of sleep apnea is central sleep apnea, which is caused by failure of stimulation of the respiratory center in the brain. Many of us have noticed irregular breathing when trying to sleep at high altitudes, such as on a hut trip at 11,000 feet. Lack of oxygen causes us to take a series of consecutive breaths, each deeper than the previous one, followed by several seconds of absent breathing as our bodies sense a low carbon dioxide level (as we take these deep breaths we blow out carbon dioxide). Due to genetics, aging, and other reasons, some people develop this irregular breathing at lower altitudes. According to Dr. Khilnani, the pulmonologist (lung specialist) who directs Valley View Hospital's Lung Center in Glenwood Springs, Colorado, central sleep apnea rarely occurs in people who live below 3,000 feet but is common in people who live above 3,000 feet. Unfortunately, central sleep apnea is under-diagnosed.

People with sleep apnea are in and out of a deep sleep during the night, unbeknownst to them. This, plus the periodic sudden drops in blood oxygen stresses their bodies, particularly their cardiovascular systems. Serious problems can result, such as: daytime sleepiness, which contributes to accidents and poor job performance; high blood pressure, especially first thing in the morning; heart failure; pulmonary hypertension; heart attacks and strokes; diabetes; "thick blood" from high red blood counts as the body tries to compensate for low oxygen at night by making more red blood cells;

cardiac rhythm disturbances such as atrial fibrillation; sudden death; depression; cognitive impairment; and erectile dysfunction.

If we doctors see someone with early morning or difficult-to-control hypertension, or if we see someone with heart irregularities, we should immediately screen for sleep apnea. Dr. Laws, the director of Valley View Hospital's Heart and Vascular Center in Glenwood Springs, Colorado, says that when patients present to him with cardiac rhythm disturbances, he always screens them for sleep apnea, and the majority of them have it. The screening test for sleep apnea is cheap and easy: an overnight oximetry, which involves wearing a monitor on your finger that records your oxygen during the night. If it is normal, sleep apnea is unlikely. If it is abnormal, the next step is an overnight sleep study. Home sleep studies are convenient, but unfortunately they aren't so good for diagnosing central sleep apnea. So, a sleep study done in a sleep lab is best.

Dr. Khilnani feels that good sleep quality is just as important for good health as good blood pressure and cholesterol, and he feels that everyone should be screened for sleep apnea. For sure get screened if you have conditions such as snoring, daytime fatigue or sleepiness, diabetes, depression, high blood pressure, diabetes, obesity, coronary artery disease, palpitations, high red blood count, ED, depression, or cognitive decline.

Treatment consists of: first of all avoiding sleep aids such as Ambien, narcotics, and more than minimal alcohol (these all depress respirations). Weight loss helps obstructive sleep apnea in obese people. Some dentists are trained in oral appliances, which can sometimes help OSA sufferers. The standard treatment for obstructive and mixed sleep apnea is CPAP (continuous positive airway pressure), which involves wearing a mask over your nose at night, with a constant airflow that pushes air past upper airway obstruction. Most although not all people tolerate CPAP, and almost all who do are surprised at how much better they sleep and at how much better they feel during the day. CPAP doesn't always work for central sleep apnea sufferers, in which case moving to a lower altitude is the answer.

THE IMPORTANCE OF ADEQUATE SLEEP

In the previous health tip I discussed one of the common causes of poor sleep: obstructive sleep apnea. However, there are many other reasons that a large percentage of Americans don't get enough sleep:

Studies show that for optimal mental and physical health, adults should get 7–8 hours of good sleep and children, including teenagers, about 10 hours. Too many of us are not achieving this, and here are some of the reasons:

- Many people work too hard and therefore stay up too late and/or get up too early.
- We get stimulated in the evening by computer and TV screens and other sources of bright light.
- Alcohol, tobacco, and caffeine interfere with sleep.
- People with depression or anxiety often have difficulty falling asleep or have early-morning awakening.
- Older men with prostate trouble often have to get up at night to urinate several times (some women too), which disrupts sleep.

Inadequate sleep can lead to poor job or school performance, auto accidents, high blood pressure, cardiovascular disease (e.g. people who get 6 or fewer or 9 or more hours of sleep a night have a significantly increased stroke risk), diabetes (from increased levels of stress hormones such as cortisol), irritability, and depression.

Here are some tips for good sleep hygiene:

- Your bedroom should be used only for sleep and sex and should be quiet, cool, and completely dark.
- Go to bed at a reasonable hour and at about the same time every night, and plan on sleeping at least 7 hours.
- Don't eat within at least 3 hours of bedtime.
- Avoid caffeine of any kind.
- Get at least 30 minutes of aerobic exercise daily such as brisk walking, but try not to do it late in the day (exercise is a stimulant).
- Alcohol helps people fall asleep but within a few hours the "rebound effect"

SLEEP

awakens them, so avoid it within 3 hours of bedtime, and stick to the recommended maximum (1 drink a day for women, 2 for men, a drink = 4 oz. of wine or 12 of beer or 1 of hard alcohol).

- Do not use a computer, a smart phone, or watch TV, and avoid all other bright lights, for 1 hour prior to bedtime. Do something such as read, with a dim light, which helps stimulate melatonin and gets your brain ready for sleep. Don't go in your bathroom right before bed and turn on bright lights to brush your teeth, because that just stimulates you again, so get a dimmer on your light switch.
- If you just can't sleep, don't lie there watching the clock, but get up and read in dim light for a while.
- If you have depression or anxiety, discuss treatment with your PCP or a psychiatrist.
- If you are getting up at night to urinate, avoid all fluids after your evening meal, and if the problem doesn't resolve, talk to your PCP or a urologist about treatment options.
- Consider a meditation class.

Sleeping medications can be helpful for some people, but some are addictive and must be used with care. Sedating anti-depressants such as Remeron (take at bedtime) and trazodone (take an hour before bedtime with a small snack) can be helpful and are not addictive.

"While heroin and cocaine and tobacco and every drug and junk food
cause dopamine release, there are healthier ways
that you can put this into your life.
And the three big ones are intimacy, physical activity ... and music."

– Neal Barnard, M.D.

SMOKING

ADVERSE HEALTH EFFECTS FROM SMOKING

Humans have been smoking for thousands of years, but it wasn't until the 1920s that scientists in Germany found a link between smoking and lung cancer. Over subsequent decades, the evidence that smoking causes health problems became overwhelming. The percentage of people in developed countries who smoke has been dropping since the 1960s, but the percentage is increasing in developing countries.

Unfortunately, 15 percent of Americans still smoke (about 36.5 million), and smoking is the most common cause of preventable death. Tobacco smoke contains over 5,000 identified chemicals, so it's not surprising that it has many adverse health effects.

The most common cause of death in the U.S. is cardiovascular disease—heart attacks and strokes. Our arteries are lined by a delicate organ called the endothelium. Smoking inflames the endothelium and causes it to thicken and eventually to form plaque (hardening of the arteries). When plaque becomes inflamed—one of the causes being smoking—it can rupture, resulting in a heart attack or stroke. Smoking can also affect the arteries in other parts of the body, causing conditions such as peripheral vascular disease (blockages in the leg arteries) and E.D.

Cigarette smoke contains a myriad of carcinogens. Nine out of 10 deaths from lung cancer in the U.S. are attributable to smoking, and lung cancer now causes more deaths in women than breast cancer. Smokers are at higher risk for many other cancers as well: bladder; blood (leukemia); cervix; colon and rectal; kidney; voice box; liver; mouth, throat and tongue; pancreas; stomach. If everyone in America stopped smoking, 1 out of 3 cancer deaths would be prevented.

Smoking also damages and destroys the delicate air sacs in the lungs, known as alveoli, resulting in emphysema, which leads to constant need for supplemental oxygen and a slow death. Smoking causes premature aging, affecting all our organs including our skin (premature wrinkling). It increases the risk of cataracts, macular degeneration, diabetes, and rheumatoid arthritis. It also harms immune function and contributes to infertility. In pregnant women it contributes to premature births, low birth weight, and cleft lip and palate. It is one of the causes of sudden infant death syndrome.

Smoking is not only bad for the people who smoke, but also for the people around them. If you were raised in a household with people who smoked, your risk is increased for several of the above conditions.

Smoking raises levels of dopamine and endorphins, making it very addictive. It's certainly best not to start smoking in the first place, but if you do smoke, it is possible to quit, and many people do. Certain prescriptions such as bupropion help, and there are helpful sites on the Internet such as Quit Colorado. Smokeless tobacco (chewing tobacco) has many of the same adverse health effects as cigarettes, and e-cigarettes have their own set of problems.

There are many similarities between the fight against Big Tobacco years ago and the current fight against Big Food, such as:

- As the science linking tobacco and disease became more overwhelming, the tobacco companies tried to deny the evidence and sow seeds of doubt on the science. Currently, food companies use the same tactics.
- Tobacco companies came up with unhelpful gimmicks such as filters and low tar cigarettes and even organic tobacco. Currently, food companies are coming up with gimmicks like "Fruit Loops now contain fiber," and "organic cane sugar."
- For years doctors didn't get that smoking was bad (remember the ad: "most doctors smoke Camels"?), but eventually they did get it, and virtually no doctors smoke these days. Currently most doctors don't get unhealthy eating and its connection to disease, but hopefully, they will.

"The people who eat the most animal protein have the most heart disease, cancer and diabetes."

– T. Colin Campbell, PhD

THE LOW-DOWN ON VITAMIN D

Vitamins are defined as organic substances occurring in many foods in small amounts that are necessary for the normal metabolic functioning of the body. Vitamin D is one of the fat-soluble vitamins. Our bodies can't manufacture vitamins but can manufacture hormones, and some experts feel that vitamin D should be classified as a hormone rather than a vitamin because our bodies manufacture it when exposed to the sun.

"Current Medical Diagnosis and Treatment 2016" notes that vitamin D deficiency "is increasing throughout the world as a result of diminished exposure to sunlight caused by urbanization, automobile and public transportation, modest clothing, and sunscreen use." Defining vitamin D deficiency can be confusing due to two ways of measuring levels: nmol/liter and ng/ml (e.g. 112 nmol/liter is the same as 50 ng/ml). The latter is the way levels are usually reported and is what will be used here. Significant vitamin D deficiency is defined as a level less than 20 ng/ml and this occurs in 29 percent of postmenopausal American women and 25 percent of American men over age 65. Severe deficiency is defined as a level less than 10 ng/ml and is present in 3.5 percent of Americans.

Almost all cells, organs, and tissues in our bodies have vitamin D receptors, and vitamin D can also turn on hundreds of genes. Over the years, vitamin D supplementation has been touted as a panacea for all sorts of health problems, but according to Dr. Greger's website *nutritionfacts.org*, better studies done in the last few years have discounted many of these claims. Here's what the current science tells us about vitamin D deficiency:

- Vitamin D promotes calcium absorption by the intestines, and also stimulates the activity of bone-forming cells called osteoblasts. Deficiency can cause osteoporosis and osteomalacia, which, like osteoporosis, causes brittle bones and fractures, but is not exactly the same as osteoporosis. In children, with developing bones, osteomalacia is called rickets, which can result in permanent skeletal deformities.
- There are vitamin D receptors in our muscles and nervous systems including our brains, but as we age the number of receptors decreases. Elderly people

with low vitamin D levels are more apt to suffer falls, due to muscle weakness and balance problems.

- Vitamin D boosts our immune system, and people with low D levels have an increased incidence of respiratory infections.
- Low vitamin D levels are associated with increased all-cause mortality (i.e. you live longer if you maintain normal vitamin D levels).
- Vitamin D helps fight inflammation. Asthma, ulcerative colitis, and Crohn's Disease, all inflammatory diseases, improve and in some cases even go into remission once D levels have normalized.
- According to Dr. Fuhrman, author of *Eat to Live* and other books, "Vitamin D regulates several genes and cellular processes related to cancer progression." People with low levels of D are more apt to get several cancers including breast and colon, and once they get cancer it is more likely to progress.

What are normal levels? Dr. Greger points out that the cradle of civilization was in equatorial Africa, "when people were running around outside naked." Vitamin D levels in African tribes living traditional lifestyles are around 50. Breast milk lacks vitamin D, and therefore breast-fed babies are given D supplements, which doesn't make sense from an evolutionary point of view. But if a breastfeeding mother's D level is 50 or greater, her breast milk does contain vitamin D. So while some guidelines say we should shoot for levels of D greater than 30, most of the science points to levels of 50 or more as ideal.

How much D should people take to achieve levels of 50 or above? For most people, 2,000 units a day achieves optimal D levels, with some caveats:

- Vitamin D is stored in fat, so obese people need to take 4,000 u a day to achieve optimal levels.
- Absorption is hampered in the elderly, so the American Geriatrics Society recommends 4,000 u in people 65 and older.
- The type of vitamin D you should take is D3, which is what your body makes when exposed to sunlight; versus D2 present in yeast and mushrooms, which isn't as effective.
- D is absorbed better if taken with a meal that contains some fat, such as nuts and seeds.
- The practice of taking very high doses (e.g. 50,000 u) intermittently is now frowned upon, because the very high levels that result can cause problems.

How about just getting sun exposure rather than taking a supplement? The problem is that sun ages your skin and causes skin cancer. When outside you should cover up and apply sunscreen to exposed areas of your skin such as your face, but this interferes with vitamin D production. Tanning booths have the same problems as sun exposure, and aren't very effective in vitamin D production anyway.

Should everyone have their vitamin D levels tested? Most guidelines don't recommend this because:

- Almost all Americans are lower than optimal in vitamin D.
- Most insurance companies and Medicare won't cover the test when coded as a screen.
- The test for vitamin D is done on a blood sample, and is not a very accurate test in that a lot of variation can occur between labs and even on the same sample tested repeatedly in the same lab.
- Vitamin D is inexpensive and has no side effects except in very high doses, such as 10,000 units a day, which can result in dangerously high blood levels.

*"Everything in food works together
to create health or disease."*

– T. Colin Campbell, PhD

BEWARE OF B12 DEFICIENCY

Vitamins are substances that the body can't make and that are necessary in trace amounts for normal metabolic functioning. Vitamin B12 (cobalamin) is a water-soluble vitamin (as opposed to fat-soluble). Unlike other vitamins, which are made by plants (vitamin D is an exception because it is produced by exposure to sunlight), B12 comes from bacteria in dirt. Animals eat food that contains dirt, and B12 is stored in their livers and muscles. B12 also ends up in eggs and dairy. The average adult needs 2.3 micrograms of B12 a day, which is adsorbed in the lower part of the small intestine (ileum). Intrinsic factor, made by parietal cells in the stomach, is necessary for absorption.

B12 is involved in every cell in the human body and in particular it is necessary for brain, nervous system, and red blood cell health. Deficiency in B12 can result in the following health problems:

- Anemia associated with abnormally large red blood cells
- Fatigue
- Numbness and tingling in hands and feet and poor balance (both of which can be irreversible)
- Poor memory, depression, and even psychosis
- Elevated homocysteine (a risk factor for cardiovascular disease)

For the most part, people who eat animal products do not experience B12 deficiency. However, the following conditions can result in deficiency, even if intake is adequate:

- Pernicious anemia (which is an autoimmune disease that destroys the intrinsic factor necessary for B12 absorption)
- Obesity surgery such as stomach stapling, and other GI tract surgery involving the stomach or small intestine
- Celiac and severe Crohn's disease
- The commonly-used diabetic drug metformin
- Drugs that prevent secretion of stomach acid taken for more than two years (PPIs such as Nexium and Prilosec; H2 blockers such as Pepcid and Zantac)
- Advanced age: people 65 and older don't absorb B12 as well

In addition, a vegan lifestyle can result in deficiency. People often ask me why, if plant-based nutrition is a "natural" diet, they have to take a B12 supplement. The answer is that we don't eat as much dirt, with B12-produced in bacteria, as we did when the human genome was evolving. For example, our water is treated (which is a good thing in that we don't get cholera or giardia), and our produce is often pre-washed.

How do you tell if you are deficient in B12? If you have any of the symptoms of B12 deficiency noted above, if your red blood cells are abnormally large, or if you have any of the above risk factors for deficiency, you should have a blood test done to check your level of B12. A more accurate test is a serum methylmalonic acid.

Deficiency is treated with supplements. For the most part, oral supplements are sufficient:—1,000 mcg. of B12 a day. In rare situations such as celiac disease or severe Crohn's disease, injections are necessary. To prevent deficiency, all vegans should supplement with 250 micrograms a day of B12 (cyanocobalamin), which is inexpensive and which you can buy at any drug store in pill form (sublingual preparations offer no advantage). People 65 and older should take 1,000 micrograms a day. It is especially important that vegan women who are pregnant take a supplement to ensure that the growing fetus gets adequate B12. Unlike other vitamins, you can't get too much vitamin B12 with oral supplementation because you can only absorb a certain amount.

Years ago doctors would give B12 injections to patients who complained of feeling tired. However, this practice is a bad idea. There are many causes of feeling tired, and B12 deficiency is an uncommon one. So, if you feel tired, you need a workup to see what the cause is and then you should be treated appropriately.

Switching from a meat-based to a plant-based diet would do more to curb and reverse global warming than any other initiative."

– T. Colin Campbell, PhD

DON'T OMIT OMEGA-3

There are healthy and unhealthy fats. Unfortunately, the S.A.D. (Standard American Diet) contains too little of the former and too much of the latter.

Unhealthy fats include saturated fats, found primarily in animal products (meat, dairy, eggs) but also in coconut and palm products and added oils. Trans fats, also known as partially hydrogenated fats, are found primarily in snack and fried foods, but some occur naturally in meat. Saturated and trans fats are clearly linked to obesity, diabetes, heart disease, and cancer.

The biochemistry of healthy fats is rather complex, but here's the simplified version:

- There are two "essential" fats, meaning that our bodies can't make them from scratch and we must get the building blocks from food. Our bodies can make other "non-essential" fats from the two essential fats.
- One of the essential fats is alpha-linolenic acid (ALA), an omega-3 fat, which our bodies convert to EPA and DHA, the latter being particularly important for brain health.
- The second essential fat is the omega-6 linolenic acid, which our bodies convert to arachidonic acid, too much of which causes inflammation.
- The building blocks for omega-3 are found in small amounts in several green vegetables, beans, and fruit. They are found in larger amounts in walnuts, seeds, and flax.
- The building blocks for omega-6 are found in small amounts in certain vegetables and seeds, but in concentrated amounts in oils made from these vegetables and seeds such as safflower and sunflower and corn oil and even olive oil (read Dr. Ornish's book *The Spectrum*).
- Optimal health results when the omega-6 to omega-3 ratio is 1:1 or at most 2:1.
- Unfortunately, the average American has a ratio between 10:1 to 30:1.

High levels of omega-6 and not enough omega-3 can result in:
- Dementia including Alzheimer's

- Heart disease
- Strokes
- Autoimmune diseases
- Depression
- Increased risk for cancer

Why not get already-made omega-3 from fatty fish (salmon, sardines, mackerel, herring, tuna, trout) or fish oil? Fish is an animal protein, which results in health problems not associated with plant protein. Furthermore, essentially all fish and other seafood, as well as fish oil, have worrisome levels of toxins such as PCBs and heavy metals. To avoid high levels of omega-6, avoid or at least cut down on added oils. To raise omega-3 levels eat the following every day:

- Ground flaxseed, 1 to 2 tablespoonfuls
- Walnuts, 12 halves.
- Soybeans or tofu 1.5 cup
- For genetic reasons, some people may not convert enough of the omega-3 building blocks to EPA and DHA. So if you don't eat fish, to ensure brain health it's wise to take 250–450 mg. a day of vegan algae-derived omega 3, which is free of contaminants. This is available at Vitamin Cottage (get the most cost-effective brand) and at *www.DrFuhrman.com*.

There is an inexpensive blood test available through some labs including the Cleveland Heart Lab that checks your omega-6 to omega-3 ratio.

*"You don't get permanently well
unless you permanently change the way you live."*

– Joel Fuhrman, M.D.

SUPPLEMENTS

CONCERNS ABOUT SUPPLEMENTS

There's no question that pharmaceuticals have their problems, although if you get pneumonia, depression, heart failure, and many other conditions you will be glad we have them. Big Pharma is easy to dislike, because among other things their main motive is profits rather than our health, and they rip people off when they can (for example, Viagra costs $40 a pill in the U.S. when the generic is a few dollars elsewhere). Some 106,000 people die from adverse reactions to drugs in the U.S. every year, making that the 4th leading cause of death. On the other hand, the FDA closely controls pharmaceuticals, which must be proven to be effective and to be relatively safe before they can be sold, and literature on possible adverse reactions must accompany each prescription that leaves the pharmacy.

However, supplements have their problems as well. When a patient makes an appointment to see me, I ask them to bring in everything they're taking. I'm always amazed when they start out by telling me they are against taking any medications, but they bring in a bag full of different supplements, some of them often expensive. Here are the problems:

- The supplement industry is a 36-billion dollar industry, and whenever money is involved, dishonesty and corruption often occur.
- In spite of what the supplement manufacturers would like you to believe, there is minimal oversight. An issue of *the American Family Physician* journal points out that "the Dietary Supplement Health and Education Act of 1994 made supplement manufacturers responsible for ensuring that their products are safe, essentially using an honor system" and "that manufacturers do not need FDA approval before selling their product." Would you trust the pharmaceutical industry to use the honor system?
- Therefore, supplements don't have to be proven to be safe or effective, often don't contain what the label says, and sometimes have dangerous contaminants. For example, Consumer's Report found heavy metals including lead and arsenic in several powdered protein supplements and noted that "you don't need the extra protein or the heavy metals" in these products. An article in the *New England Journal* pointed out that there are some 23,000 ER visits a year

related to dietary supplements, with over 2,000 hospitalizations. Liver toxicity, which can lead to liver failure and even death, can rarely occur with certain pharmaceuticals but also from certain supplements, either from the supplements themselves or from contaminants. People who eat a diet high in antioxidant vitamins (fruits and vegetables and whole grains) have better health and longer lives, but vitamin A and E in pill form raise risk for early death. Calcium in vegetables such as kale, and fruit such as figs and oranges, promotes strong bones, but calcium supplements increase the risk of heart attacks, per the book *Beat The Heart Attack Gene*. Folate in vegetables helps prevent cancer, while folic acid pills increase cancer risk.

- Due to lack of oversight, false claims are often made by supplement manufacturers. In his book *How Not to Die,* Michael Greger notes that pyramid-like multilevel supplement companies "espouse all sorts of health claims" and that a public health review found that such studies often seemed "deliberately created for marketing purposes" and were bogus.
- Many dietary supplements interact with other supplements and with pharmaceuticals, including Coumadin.

People often tell me they don't want to take a statin but would rather take "something natural like red yeast rice." I tell them that just because something is natural doesn't mean it's healthy (arsenic and lead for example). Toxic contaminants were found in red yeast rice from China. Furthermore, the only reason this product lowers cholesterol a little is that it contains a natural statin, lovastatin—the first statin that came on the market 25 or so years ago under the brand name Mevacor. So I suggest that they take the actual drug, because we can be sure it contains what's on the label and doesn't have impurities. But I also tell them what's even better is to go on a plant-based, whole foods diet, which we know is the most effective and for sure the safest way to prevent and reverse cardiovascular disease and to prevent cancer.

SUPPLEMENTS

SHOULD YOU TAKE SUPPLEMENTS?

Vitamins and minerals are substances necessary in trace amounts for normal metabolic functioning of cells in the human body. With two exceptions, vitamins are made by plants; although because animals eat plants vitamins are present in some animal products.

The two exceptions are vitamin B12—made by bacteria in dirt—and vitamin D, produced in our skin when it's exposed to sun. Due to treated water and pre-washed produce these days, vegans may not get enough B12, which can lead to neurologic problems, so they should take a 1,000 mcg. B12 supplement daily. All seniors should take B12 as well, even if their diet is meat-based, because many elderly people don't absorb B12 well. Vitamin D is made by our skin when exposed to the sun. The human genome evolved over millions of years in equatorial Africa, when pre-humans and humans were running around mainly naked. Most Americans are D deficient, and should take a supplement daily: 1,000 I.U. a day for adults, 2,000 if 65 or older (if you want to be scientific about it, have your blood level checked).

How about minerals and other vitamins? They are clearly important for optimal health. In the distant past people suffered from diseases such as scurvy caused by lack of vitamin C, and beriberi due to deficiency of vitamin B1 (thiamine). In our part of the world, diseases due to deficiency of vitamins other than D and B12 are rare now.

In Western societies we like to practice what T. Colin Campbell, PhD (featured in the documentary *Forks Over Knives*, author of *The China Study* and *Whole*) calls "reductionism." Different foods have been shown to cause certain health benefits, and we like to find the "magic bullet" responsible for these benefits, put it in a pill or capsule, market it and make millions in profits. The problem is that nutrition isn't that simple. There are thousands of vitamins, co-vitamins, and other nutrients in various unprocessed plant foods, many of which remain unknown, and many of which work synergistically. As Dr. Esselstyn (also featured in *Forks Over Knives*, author of *Prevent and Reverse Heart Disease*) puts it, if we eat a "symphony of plant-based food" our bodies have an amazing way of taking out what we need.

You cannot get the same thing in pill or capsule form, plus we didn't evolve to be able to handle the large doses of vitamins we get in pill form. For example, people who eat plants rich in vitamin E have less heart disease, but high doses of vitamin E in pill form increase the risk of heart attacks. Vitamin A-containing food helps prevent cancer, but high doses in pill form increase the risk of lung cancer in smokers. Calcium supplements increase the risk of heart disease. Joel Fuhrman, M.D., author of several books including *Eat to Live*, notes that folic acid, the synthetic form of folate, is added to food and used in vitamin supplements. Whole foods with natural folate prevent disease, whereas "evidence suggests that folic acid supplementation may significantly increase the risk of cancer."

Regarding minerals, in his book *Power Foods For The Brain*, Neal Barnard, M.D. points out that:

- The amount of copper we need is 0.9 mg. which can easily be obtained by eating greens, nuts, whole grains, and mushrooms. There is evidence that larger doses from supplements or from cookware may contribute to Alzheimer's.
- Daily iron requirements can be met by eating greens, beans, whole grains, and dried fruits, but too much from supplements and cookware may contribute to Alzheimer's. (Note that women with heavy menses might need iron supplements if their red blood count is low.)
- We need 8 to 11 mg. of zinc daily, with healthy sources being oatmeal, whole-grain bread, brown rice, peanuts, beans, nuts, peas, and sesame seeds. Too much in pill form may contribute to Alzheimer's.

Many studies have proven that multi-vitamin and mineral supplements are not beneficial and may even be harmful. Yet 1/3 of Americans spend billions of dollars on them. Here's the bottom line:

- Vegan and elderly Americans are at risk for B12 deficiency and should supplement. Most Americans need to supplement with vitamin D3.
- We evolved to get other vitamins and trace minerals in our food—by eating a variety of vegetables, fruit, and whole grains—not in pill or liquid form.
- If you eat animal products, eat more plant-based foods as well.
- You cannot get from pills what you can get by eating a healthy diet.

A couple of caveats:

- We should avoid salt because it harms the endothelial lining of blood vessels and eventually leads to high blood pressure. Years ago, in order to prevent goiters, guidelines were put in place to add iodine to commercial salt. If you don't eat salt you can get iodine by eating seaweed every day, by eating Eden brand canned beans (which contain a tiny bit of kelp), or by taking a 150 microgram supplement of iodine a day (especially important in pregnant and breastfeeding women).
- If you are plant-based and want more details about vitamins and minerals, Dr. Greger (*nutritionfacts.org*, author of *How Not to Die*) recommends a reference book by "the preeminent dietitians" Brenda Davis and Vesanto Melina called *The Complete Guide to Adopting a Plant-Based Diet*.

SUPPLEMENTS

FOUNTAIN OF YOUTH?
TWEAK YOUR TELOMERES

Each human cell has 23 chromosomes, each made up of two strands of DNA. At the tip of the chromosomes are caps called telomeres that keep the DNA from unraveling and are analogous to the plastic tips at each end of your shoelaces. As soon as you're born, telomeres gradually shorten. As they shorten, you age, and when they're gone cells die, and eventually you die.

A few years ago scientists were studying the oldest organisms on the planet, bristlecone pines in California, one of which is 4,800 years old and still going strong. Their investigation led them to an enzyme in the roots of bristlecones that rebuilds telomeres. The scientists named the enzyme telomerase, and the enzyme was subsequently found to be present in human cells as well. Levels of telomerase can be measured, and are related to the health and length of your telomeres, and therefore your health and the length of your life.

Although this is still evolving science, studies done so far show that the following hasten telomere shortening and therefore aging in humans:
- Smoking (cigarettes triples the rate of loss of telomere length)
- Consumption of refined grains, soda, meat, fish, and dairy
- Chronic emotional stress (We've all seen people under chronic stress who age rapidly. Dr. Dean Ornish did a study of mothers of chronically ill children who aged by 10 years based on telomere length, compared to a control group.)
- Inflammation

Here's what has been shown to preserve telomere length and to even repair damage once it occurs:
- Antioxidant-rich foods such as fruit and vegetables are more effective than anything else in preserving telomere length.
- Dr. Ornish showed that stress reduction through activities such as mindfulness meditation increase telomerase levels and lengthen shortened telomeres, which he discusses in his book *The Spectrum*.
- Regular exercise also helps.

If you want to stack the deck in your favor to increase your chance of living a long, healthy life, do what it takes to keep your telomeres long. To find out more, go to Dr. Greger's website *nutritionfacts.org* and search telomeres, or read *The Spectrum.*

TELOMERES

"A good diet is the most powerful weapon
we have against disease and sickness."

– T. Colin Campbell, PhD

PLANT-BASED, WHOLE (UNPROCESSED) FOOD, MODERATELY LOW-FAT DIET, WHICH SCIENCE SUPPORTS AS BEING THE HEALTHIEST

Patient Handout

DON'T EAT

Don't eat the following, all of which are calorie-dense; have few micronutrients; lack fiber and have been shown to contribute to obesity, high cholesterol, heart attacks, strokes, type 2 diabetes, hypertension, inflammatory and autoimmune diseases, dementia, osteoporosis and many types of cancer:

- Meat, including chicken
- Dairy, including cheese and yogurt
- Eggs
- Seafood: animal protein, contaminants such as PCBs and heavy metals
- Oils, including coconut and olive (Stir fry with water, veggie broth, vinegar or wine For baking substitute unsweetened apple sauce and/or ground flaxseed. Use vinegar for salad dressing.)
- Processed food such as white bread, white pasta (use a spiralizer to make your own veggie "pasta"), white flour tortillas, white rice (Avoid more than occasional rice anyway due to arsenic contamination.)
- Sugar (Check the food label and see what the serving size is, then look at grams of sugar. Four grams is a teaspoon.)
- Salt—maximum salt intake should be 1,500 mg. a day (As long as you don't have chronic kidney disease, use NoSalt salt—potassium chloride, found in salt section at grocery store—instead of sodium chloride.)

DO EAT

Do eat the following every day, because they have a high nutrient per calorie ratio, have antioxidants and phytonutrients that prevent and reverse almost all of the chronic diseases associated with the S.A.D. (Standard American Diet). Dr. Greger, in his book

How Not to Die, explains his daily dozen: beans, berries, other fruits, cruciferous vegetables, greens, other vegetables, flaxseeds, nuts, spices, whole grains, beverages, exercise.

- "Eat the rainbow." Foods with intense color (e.g. greens, peppers, red cabbage, red onions, berries, yams) or intense flavor (herbs and spices) are particularly healthful. Mushrooms and cauliflower are exceptions, being non-colorful yet healthy vegetables.
- Main emphasis should be on a variety of vegetables daily, including green leafy veggies; cruciferous veggies (e.g. broccoli, cabbage, collards, kale). Eat at least some of your veggies raw, as in salads.
- Daily legumes: beans, lentils, chick peas (garbanzo beans). After 2 weeks gassiness and bloating resolves if you stick with it. Most people tolerate edamame best.
- Whole grains such as rolled or steel-cut oats, multigrain hot cereal; black ("forbidden") rice, which is healthier than red followed by brown rice; Dave's Killer or low-sodium Ezekiel bread (at Whole Foods and Vitamin Cottage in the cooler).
- Check food labels, if total the total carbs: fiber ratio is 5:1 or less, the product has lots of whole grains and fiber (multiply the fiber number by 5, and that number should be greater than the number for total carbs). Beware of misleading advertising on bread wrappers and cereal boxes claiming "whole wheat" when it really isn't.
- Herbs and spices, including 1/4 teaspoon of turmeric a day (buy in bulk at Vitamin Cottage).
- Fruit, including citrus and non-citrus (pears, plums, apples, etc.). Berries are intensely colored and especially nutritious. Frozen organic berries, available at Vitamin Cottage, are just as nutritious as fresh. You can find cost-effective frozen organic blueberries at Costco.
- Seeds: Sprinkle raw, unsalted pumpkin and sunflower seeds on your salad.
- Beverages: Tap water is fine. The healthiest drink is hot or iced berry tea with hibiscus as the first ingredient, which you can find at City Market. Green tea is second best but has some caffeine.
- Nuts: Eat a handful of raw, unsalted nuts every day. Walnuts have the healthiest ratio of good to bad fats, followed by almonds and pecans and peanuts.
- Eat 1–2 tablespoons of ground flax seeds a day. Refrigerate.

SUPPLEMENTS

Supplements, take only these, (you'll be getting everything else you need the way you're meant to—through the food you eat):

- VERY IMPORTANT, take 1,000 mcg of B12 daily.
- Take 250–450 mg. a day of vegan, algae-derived omega-3 daily. Available at Vitamin Cottage (ask for an inexpensive brand) or get it through Dr. Fuhrman's website, *www.Dr.Fuhrman.com*.
- Most Americans are low in vitamin D so take 1,000 units a day of D3, 2,000 units a day if 65 or older.

SNACKS

- Rip Esselstyn's Engine 2 Plant Strong products at Whole Foods are healthy, including hummus w/o added oil (dip carrot in it) and crackers.
- Another good snack for both adults and children are organic shelled edamame, available at Vitamin Cottage and Whole Foods.

DESSERT

- Slice up and freeze bananas. After dinner put a few slices in a bowl along with berries, add a small amount of Bob's Red Mill Old County Style muesli and unsweetened almond milk.
- Eat dessert right after dinner, so your body only has to secrete one insulin bolus.

BREAKFAST

- Buy bulk steel cut oats at Whole Foods. Once a week, put in a pan with water and bring to a boil, let it set for a few hours and it's done. Keep in the fridge and every morning get a bowl of it out and heat in a microwave. Add cinnamon, a handful of frozen edamame, 1–2 tablespoons of ground flax, your handful of walnuts for the day, berries, raisins, 1/4 teaspoon of turmeric, then some unsweetened almond or soy milk.
- If you need more, add 2 pieces of low sodium Ezekiel bread, put unsweetened apple sauce on it and sprinkle cinnamon on it.
- On Sundays, make pancakes out of buckwheat and garbanzo bean flour, add walnuts, pumpkin spice and unsweetened almond milk. Put unsweetened apple sauce and berries on the pancakes.

EXERCISE

- At least 30 min. of aerobic exercise a day, hard enough so you can talk but not sing. If 40 or over, also do strength training for 20 min. twice a week.
- If you have a desk job, use a standup desk or move about every 30 minutes.

DVDs

- *Forks Over Knives** is an excellent, 90-min. documentary. Available on YouTube and Netflix.
- Dietitian Jeff Novick's Fast Food DVD series is helpful if you don't like to cook and just want the cheapest, easiest way to make healthy meals.

BOOKS

- *Prevent and Reverse Heart Disease* by Caldwell Esselstyn, M.D. — 100 pages of easy reading followed by recipes. Keep in mind that Dr. E. is trying to reverse heart disease and is too hard core re. avoiding nuts and seeds for most people.
- *How Not to Die* by Michael Greger, M.D.* is a must-have. First half is about how not to die from various conditions, second half is about what we should be eating every day and why. It is 400 pages but the last quarter is references, so very evidence-based.
- If you have a family history of heart disease or have a known disease yourself, read *Beat the Heart Attack Gene* by Bale and Doneen.

COOKBOOKS

- *Oh She Glows,* by Angela Liddon (substitute unsweetened apple sauce and or ground flax seeds in recipes that call for oil)
- *Isa Does It* by Chandra Moskowitz
- *Thug Kitchen* by Matt Holloway, Michelle Davis, and Thug Kitchen
- *Forks Over Knives: The Cookbook* by Del Sroufe
- *Simply Delicious,* simple but delicious recipes by Sandy Holmes
- *How Not to Die Cookbook* by Dr. Michael Greger
- *Vegan Richa's Indian Kitchen* by Richa Hingle

WEBSITES

- Dr. Greger's *nutritionfacts.org.* Very evidence-based, and he has no ties to Big Food or Big Pharma.
You can subscribe and/or search topics.
- PCRM (Physician Committee for Responsible Medicine)* Information and recipes in 4 languages, including Spanish. It has a three-week kick-start program: *21/DayKickstart.org.*

* Available in Spanish

PATIENT HANDOUT

TIPS FOR CONVERTING TO A PLANT-BASED DIET
by Kathy Feinsinger, R.N., N.P.

The information in this health tip comes from my wife, Kathy, who is a retired nurse practitioner and an excellent cook. She developed a practical handout to give to people who want to make the transition to plant-based nutrition.

When people want to make this transition, it's important that they understand the health benefits. The following options for obtaining this information are available:

- Watch the *Forks Over Knives* documentary, available on Netflix.
- Buy *How Not to Die*, by Michael Greger, M.D. Read any chapters in the first half of the book that might apply to you (e.g. heart disease, diabetes, cancer). Then read the whole second half, about what we should be eating every day and why.
- Obtain the Plant-Based Nutrition Quick Start Guide from The Plantrician Project, *www.plantricianproject.org* (available in English and Spanish).

GENERAL SUGGESTIONS

- Remake your favorite dishes into plant-based ones.
- Set a goal of collecting 30 recipes that you can use repeatedly, on a rotational basis.
- Keep a journal of successful meals and food ideas.
- Avoid sugar (when reading food labels, 4 grams is a teaspoon). Avoid refined food (e.g. white flour, white rice, white pasta). Avoid added salt (sodium chloride)—1,500 mg. a day is the maximum safe amount for adults. Instead use potassium chloride (e.g. NoSalt salt in the salt section of the grocery store–people with chronic kidney disease should avoid potassium). For additional flavoring use herbs and spices. Avoid added oil including olive oil—replace with ground flaxseeds and/or unsweetened apple sauce.
- To plan meals, start with a base of a grain, whole grain pasta, polenta, beans, lentils, gnocchi, mushrooms, tofu, spaghetti squash, or multigrain wraps.
- Consider ethnic dishes: Mexican, Indian, Asian, Italian, Middle Eastern.
- Spend an afternoon making veggie burgers, falafel, calzones, casseroles, soups, etc. to freeze.

- A pressure cooker or the new "instant pot" are time-savers for cooking legumes, grains, and soups.

COOKING TIPS

- Toast grains in a skillet over medium heat for 3–4 minutes to bring out flavor.
- Replace oil in salad dressing with fruit juice, unsweetened applesauce, or apple cider reduction.
- You don't need oil to sauté—use veggie broth, water, or leftover white wine instead.
- Consider stuffing peppers, mushrooms, zucchini, or tomatoes (Kathy's favorite is poblano peppers).
- Become familiar with nutritional yeast—it has a nutty flavor and is a staple in plant-based cooking.
- Substitute mashed, cooked chickpeas in your favorite recipe for egg or tuna salad—use vegan mayo called Veganaise.
- Baked sweet or purple potatoes are a nutritious, inexpensive, easy side dish.
- Enjoy sauces with your food; hot sauces, Veganaise, guacamole, nut-based sauces such as cashew, hummus without added oil, tapenade, salsa, teriyaki, peanut, curry, baba ghanoush, sweet and sour, soy sauce, pesto, aioli, and no-cheese-cheese sauce (in many vegan cookbooks).
- Add unsalted nuts and/or seeds, dried or fresh fruit, leftover beans, or grains to your salads.
- When making soup use veggie broth without added salt—toss in a cube of veggie bouillon and a thumb-sized piece of kombu.
- Cruciferous vegetables (cauliflower, broccoli, cabbage, kale, bok choy, brussels sprouts, etc.) have a potent cancer-fighting micronutrient, the release of which requires an enzyme that is destroyed by cooking. So, eat some raw cruciferous veggies such as cauliflower or broccoli before eating cooked ones. Another strategy is to chop up cruciferous veggies you're planning on cooking 45 minutes prior to cooking; this releases the enzyme which can then do its job before cooking begins. Another strategy is to add horse radish, which is a cruciferous vegetable, to the cooked ones.

THE FREEZER IS YOUR FRIEND

- When cooking items such as grains, beans, soups, and vegan chili, always make extra and freeze it.
- Keep your freezer stocked with store-bought items such as corn, peas, onions, breads, seeds, nuts, and organic edamame, which make food preparation easier.

- Buy lemons on sale, squeeze them and freeze the juice in ice cube trays. Do the same thing with veggie broth, which you can use later when cooking.
- Freeze sliced bananas to use for smoothies and desserts.

MENU IDEAS FOR DINNER PARTIES

- Salads, such as niçoise. You can add tuna, salmon, or shrimp for non-vegans.
- Kebabs—lots of flexibility in providing for vegans and non-vegans.
- Vegan stir fry, curries (avoid ghee and coconut), lasagna.
- Risotto—try the pressure cooker recipe on the Internet.
- Tacos—a taco bar is a fun way for people to have different options to put on their tacos.
- Burritos are always popular.
- Noodle or rice bowls—have vegan and non-vegan options for people to add to their bowls (use veggie broth for the noodle bowls—non-vegans won't complain is they can put chicken, meat or fish on top).

A FEW RECIPES

- Sweet potato and black bean enchiladas—*vegetariantimes.com*, 12/20/2011
- Four grain and vegetable burritos—*myrecipes.com*
- Spinach, chickpea and squash gnocchi—*eatingwell.com*
- Black ("forbidden") rice salad with mango and peanuts—*epicurious.com*
- Vegan lasagna—*chow.com* (it's important to slice the eggplant 1/4 inches thick)
- Ginger cookies—*joyofyum.com*
- Chia pudding from *joyofyum.com* (top this with bananas foster and sprinkle granola on top)

IMPORTANT PRODUCTS TO KEEP ON HAND IN THE CUPBOARD

- Agar-agar is a plant-based thickening agent made from sea vegetables. Like gelatin—an animal-based product—it has no taste. Found in the Asian markets or in the baking section of large grocery stores. Arrowroot powder can also be used for thickening.
- Agave nectar, dates, and maple syrup are good sweeteners for baking and cooking. You end up using less than you would if using sugar because the flavors are more intense.
- Unsweetened soy, almond, hemp, and rice milk can be substituted for cows' milk—usually recipes specify which one to use, as some work better than others depending on the recipe.
- Fresh herbs are nutritious and tasty—freeze what you don't use.

- Raw, unsalted seeds are good on salads and soups. Use Pinon nuts more sparingly. Keep chia and ground flaxseeds on hand. If you don't use these items within a few days, move them to the freezer so they don't become rancid.
- Keep raisins, currents, dates and figs, grains, beans (dried and no-added-salt canned), chickpeas, and lentils on hand.
- Nutritional yeast has a rich, nutty flavor and is good for making a cheesy sauce (recipes in vegan cookbooks and websites). Try sprinkling it on popcorn, along with NoSalt salt (potassium instead of sodium) and cinnamon.
- Low sodium veggie broth and canned tomatoes.
- Unsweetened applesauce for baking and salad dressing.
- Wild rice pasta, which is more filling than regular pasta—so you eat less.
- Gnocchi is a potato dumpling and only needs some veggies and marinara sauce for a great, quick meal. Shelf-stable whole wheat gnocchi only needs to be browned, then it's ready to eat (no boiling necessary).
- Kombu is a type of sea vegetable found in Asian markets or the Asian section of large grocery stores. Use a thumb-sized piece when cooking beans, legumes, and soups to enhance flavor. A side-benefit is that it helps break down gas-causing components of beans. Kombu is a good source of omega-3 and iodine.
- Dulse is another sea vegetable that is delicious when added to soups, sandwiches, salads, and stir-fries. It can be found in the same places that kombu is found, and is a good source of iodine, vitamin B6, potassium, iron, and fiber.
- Keep a supply of dried mushrooms in your pantry, especially shitake and porcini. They need to be soaked for about an hour before cooking, and should not be eaten raw (raw mushrooms have a mild carcinogen that is destroyed by cooking). They are packed with nutrients, including vitamins, minerals, antioxidants, and cancer-fighting phytonutrients.

WEBSITES FOR VEGAN RECIPES

- *minimalistbaker.com*
- *ohsheglows.com*
- *joyofyum.com*
- *chowhound.com*
- *101cookbooks.com*
- *marthastewart.com*

VEGAN COOKBOOKS

- *Oh She Glows*
- *Isa Does It*
- *Thug Kitchen*
- *Forks Over Knives Cookbook*
- *Simply Delicious*
- *How Not to Die Cookbook*
- *Vegan Richa's Indian Kitchen*

INDEX

INDEX

INDEX

INDEX

INDEX

ABOUT THE AUTHOR

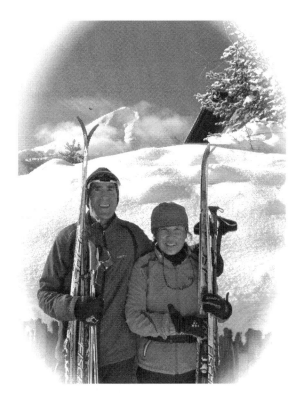

Dr. Greg and Kathy Feinsinger

Dr. Greg Feinsinger was raised in Aspen, Colorado, where his role models were his family's general practitioners. His parents always encouraged him to go into medicine, because in medicine you can be assured of helping others—the most satisfying thing in life.

He graduated from Aspen High School in 1959, and received a B.A. in political science from Oberlin College in Oberlin, Ohio, in 1963. He received his M.D. from the University of Colorado School of Medicine in Denver, in 1968, followed by a rotating internship at San Joaquin County Hospital in Stockton, California, from 1968 to 1969. From 1969 to 1971 he served in the Indian Health Service in Fort Hall, Idaho. He completed a family practice residency at Community Hospital of Sonoma County, in Santa Rosa, California, affiliated with the University of California San Francisco in 1973. The same year he joined Glenwood Medical Associates in Glenwood Springs, Colorado, where he practiced family medicine for forty-two years, retiring in 2015.

Dr. Feinsinger met his wife, Kathy, when he was a sophomore in medical school and she was a sophomore in nursing school at the University of Colorado—they were married in 1966. Kathy later worked as a nurse practitioner at Rocky Mountain Planned Parenthood for twenty-seven years. They have three grown children and eight grandchildren.

After retirement, Dr. Feinsinger started a nonprofit: Prevention and Treatment of Disease Through Nutrition. He does free consultations about heart attack prevention, nutrition, and other medical issues; promotes plant-based nutrition through lectures; is involved with a monthly plant-based potluck; and writes weekly health columns for the Glenwood *Post Independent*.

He is a Worldloppet Gold Master (completed eleven of the long version of Worldloppet Nordic ski races on three continents) and continues to run and mountain bike.